BRAIN
HACKS

BRAIN HACKS

200+ WAYS TO BOOST YOUR BRAIN POWER

ADAMS MEDIA

NEW YORK   LONDON   TORONTO   SYDNEY   NEW DELHI

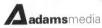

Adams Media
An Imprint of Simon & Schuster, Inc.
57 Littlefield Street
Avon, Massachusetts 02322

First Adams Media trade paperback edition FEBRUARY 2018

ADAMS MEDIA and colophon are trademarks of Simon and Schuster.

For information about special discounts for bulk purchases, please contact Simon & Schuster Special Sales at 1-866-506-1949 or business@simonandschuster.com.

The Simon & Schuster Speakers Bureau can bring authors to your live event. For more information or to book an event contact the Simon & Schuster Speakers Bureau at 1-866-248-3049 or visit our website at www.simonspeakers.com.

Interior design by Colleen Cunningham

Manufactured in the United States of America

10 9 8 7 6 5 4 3 2 1

Library of Congress Cataloging-in-Publication Data
Adams Media, (firm).
Brain hacks.
Avon, Massachusetts: Adams Media, 2018.
LCCN 2017032615 (print) | LCCN 2017041090 (ebook) | ISBN 9781507205723 (pb) | ISBN 9781507205730 (ebook)
LCSH: Mental illness--Prevention--Popular works. | Mental health--Nutritional aspects--Popular works. | Self-care, Health--Popular works.
LCC RA790 (ebook) | LCC RA790 .B73 2017 (print) | DDC 616.89/05--dc23
LC record available at https://lccn.loc.gov/2017032615

ISBN 978-1-5072-0572-3
ISBN 978-1-5072-0573-0 (ebook)

Contains material adapted from the following titles published by Adams Media, an Imprint of Simon & Schuster, Inc.: *365 Ways to Boost Your Brain Power* by Carolyn Dean, MD, Valentine Dmitriev, PhD, and Donna Raskin, copyright © 2009, ISBN 978-1-60550-060-7; *The Everything® Guide to the MIND Diet* by Christy Ellingsworth and Murdoc Khaleghi, MD, copyright © 2016, ISBN 978-1-4405-9799-2; and *The Everything® Guide to Nootropics* by Evan Brand, NTP, CPT, copyright © 2016, ISBN 978-1-4405-9131-0.

CONTENTS

INTRODUCTION

It's time to get the most out of your gray matter!

For centuries people have been looking for ways to keep their minds healthy and strong, and you can do it too. In fact, boosting your brain power has never been easier. The brain hacks in this book will help you focus longer, improve your memory, stay on your game, and keep your brain as healthy as it can be no matter your age.

You'll find more than 200 hacks—all ones you can try right away—that will help you do everything from building your memory to rejuvenating and stimulating your mind. From foods that can protect your brain's health to activities that will boost your brain power, the hacks in this book will help your brain become more fit and function better. You should see an improvement in your performance in all areas of your life, be it at work or at home.

You'll find hacks that describe what you should eat for optimum brain health, show you what activities to do (and which to avoid) to keep your brain engaged, and the best practices, according to current research, for making sure you're taking good care of those three pounds of gray matter. Whether you do one hack or all of them, this book is here to help you create a happier, healthier brain!

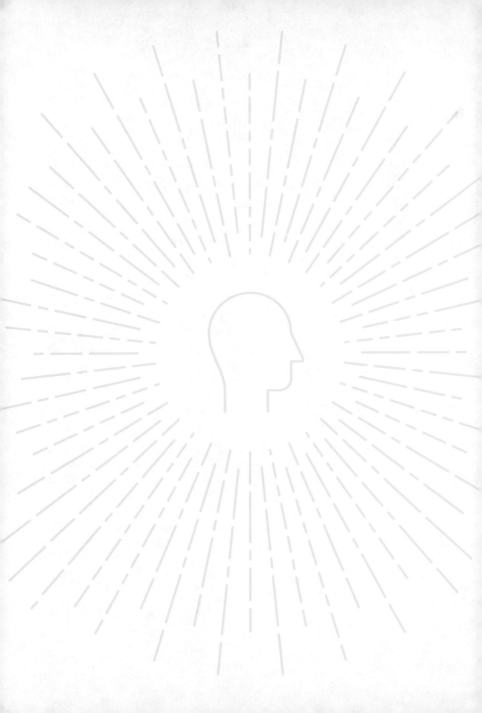

FEED YOUR BRAIN

Boost your brain power with the right food. Eat plant-based foods and healthy fats. Cut back on animal products and saturated fats (typically, solid fats like lard and butter), because saturated fats slow down your cognitive function. The nutrients found in plants, by contrast, support memory retention and help lower blood pressure (hypertension affects your brain as well as your heart). Standout stars? Beans and green, leafy vegetables.

Ten Foods to Favor
1. Beans and other legumes
2. Coconut oil
3. Fish, especially fatty fish like tuna and salmon
4. Green, leafy vegetables (e.g., spinach, kale, lettuce, and arugula)
5. Nuts, either raw or dry roasted
6. Olive oil
7. Cruciferous (cabbage family) vegetables (e.g., cauliflower)
8. Lean poultry, such as skinless chicken and ground turkey
9. Whole grains
10. Wine, either white or red (but not too much!)

Five Foods to Forget
1. Butter and margarine
2. Cheese
3. Fried foods
4. Pastries and desserts
5. Red meat, especially high-fat processed meat like bacon, sausage, and salami

According to research, the more closely you stick to a plant-based diet, the more positively you will affect your brain health.

WATCH THE ALCOHOL

Drinking too much alcohol slows your reactions, impairs your judgment, and can even cause blackouts and memory lapses—and that's just on a Friday night. In the long term, alcohol abuse can cause permanent brain damage. The National Institute of Alcohol Abuse and Alcoholism reports that long-term drinking can actually shrink your brain! It also creates problems with the structures that carry information between brain cells—making it harder for you to think and react even when you're stone-cold sober. Because heavy drinkers often have poor diets, dietary deficiencies may also harm the brain. Consume alcohol in moderation—preferably no more than two drinks per day for men and one drink per day for women.

UP YOUR OMEGA-3S

Your brain needs omega-3 fatty acids to function, but your body can't produce them. That means you have to get them from your diet. Two 2017 brain studies from the University of Illinois at Urbana-Champaign suggest that eating omega-3 fatty acids may improve memory retention and strengthen the structures responsible for fluid intelligence (the ability to solve new problems). The new research supports the idea that upping your intake of these fatty acids can slow age-related cognitive decline.

In addition, researchers at Harvard University found that omega-3 fatty acids may interfere with the brain signals that trigger the characteristic mood swings seen with bipolar disorder. If these findings hold true in future studies, omega-3 fatty acids may have implications for treating other psychiatric disorders, such as depression and schizophrenia.

Some studies have found that omega-3s can significantly decrease triglyceride levels, lower blood pressure, and reduce blood levels of homocysteine, high levels of which are associated with an increased risk of stroke, Alzheimer's disease, and other brain problems.

Foods rich in omega-3 fatty acids include:

- Flaxseed (linseed), soybean, and canola oils
- Cold-water fatty fish, like salmon, tuna, and sardines
- Certain fortified dairy and soy products (look for fortified dairy products by brand)
- Nuts, especially walnuts
- Legumes, such as pinto beans and peas

Your body needs more than one type of omega-3 fatty acid, so eat a variety of these foods every chance you get. You can also supplement with 10 grams of fish oil a day.

MAKE A TO-DO LIST

Writing a to-do list may not seem like much of a brain booster, but it is. Figuring out your priorities and filtering out the nonessentials are higher-level cognitive tasks, and practicing these skills keeps your brain in top-notch shape. Also, translating a big-picture problem or goal ("Get ready to file taxes") into its smaller tasks ("Find my W-2" and "Get recommendations for which tax software to use") is another executive function. Making a to-do list creates mental space for doing other tasks, not just remembering the various things you have to do. Plus, using a to-do list can make you feel good: one study showed that you get a little dopamine rush every time you cross a task off your to-do list (dopamine makes you feel good, elevating your mood). You should list even small tasks just for the reward of marking through them. One researcher explained that the frequency of progress is more important to your brain than how big the progress is. Practically speaking, this means crossing off "Empty the dishwasher," "Wipe the counters," and "Sweep the floor" is way more satisfying than crossing off "Clean the kitchen." (By the way, writing down something you've already done and then crossing it off creates the same happy feeling.)

STRESS LESS

Stress makes your brain think you're in danger. It responds by maintaining a high state of alertness and producing chemicals called glucocorticoids. If nothing tells your brain, "The danger has passed," those chemicals keep streaming through your blood. In effect, they become toxic to your brain. A brain on high alert is focused on survival, and thus has no time for rest and regeneration.

Stress has these key symptoms:

- Inability to relax
- Emotional instability/mood swings
- Headaches
- Sleeplessness

Stress messes with your brain by:

- Creating free radicals that kill your brain cells
- Making you forget things
- Intensifying your anxiety and irritability
- Interfering with the creation of new brain cells
- Increasing your risk for mental illness, such as depression
- Shrinking your brain, causing memory and decision-making problems
- Allowing toxins into your brain
- Escalating your likelihood of getting Alzheimer's or dementia
- Killing off brain cells prematurely

Banish stress for a healthier brain. Acknowledge when you're stressed, then resolve to take care of those problems you can (and promise yourself not to dwell on those you can't).

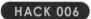

COMBAT CORTISOL

Chronic stress elevates cortisol levels, which is one of the main causes of brain cell death. A recent study found evidence of a link between the hormone cortisol and the speed of decline among Alzheimer's patients. Higher levels of cortisol correlate with shrinkage of the brain's hippocampus, which is associated with long-term memory.

Actions you take to reduce your stress, such as exercising and eating brain-healthy foods, reduce cortisol levels. In addition, fish oil supplements and an herbal supplement called ashwagandha (also known as Indian ginseng) have both been shown to help reduce cortisol levels. Prebiotic and probiotic supplements show promise of reducing cortisol levels as well.

NOSH WITH YOUR PEEPS

How many times a week do you sit down to dinner with your family? If you're like most people, maybe once or twice a week. Other times, it's likely you eat in your car, at your computer, watching television, or doing something else. But studies have shown that sitting down to dinner with your family has many benefits. People who plan and cook regular dinners eat more fruits and vegetables and get more vitamins and minerals, all of which help keep your brain healthy. In contrast, restaurant meals tend to have more calories and fat (in some cases portion sizes are double—or more—what is considered a serving).

Not only do family dinners provide your body with better fuel, they improve relationships, which are a key part of maintaining a healthy brain. Spending time together as a family helps people feel they are loved and belong. This isn't just true of children—adults have the same experience of improved relationships with other members of the family. Studies have shown that families who eat together are happier, emotionally stronger, and more resilient (better able to cope with setbacks). In one study, mothers who ate with their children were less stressed than those who did not. This was true even of mothers who worked outside the home at demanding jobs—people who you might think would experience less stress if they skipped meal planning and preparation.

FIGHT FREE RADICALS

Let's start this hack with a brief chemistry refresher. Remember how tiny particles called electrons, protons, and neutrons make up atoms? Atoms want their electrons to come in pairs, so as to stabilize themselves. Unstable atoms (or groups of atoms) have one or more unpaired electrons. In the body, these unstable atoms, called free radicals, try to complete themselves by stealing electrons from other atoms. This thievery can create a destructive chain reaction.

Your body produces some free radicals as a result of natural chemical reactions. Stress, trauma, pollution, processed foods, and drugs create others. Free radicals help your immune system do its work, but too many will damage and destroy normal healthy cells. Free radicals are thought to contribute to more than sixty different health conditions, including Alzheimer's.

To keep free radicals (sometimes called oxidants) in check, you need antioxidants, which can be found in many vitamins and minerals. Antioxidants clean up roving free radicals before they inflict damage on the brain. Also, take steps to reduce your exposure to environmental pollutants, such as pesticides, solvents, exhaust fumes, and tobacco smoke.

EAT YOUR E

Vitamin E, a natural antioxidant found in many foods, diminishes the damage caused by free radicals. Some evidence suggests that free radical damage to the neurons (nerve cells) is at least partially responsible for the development of Alzheimer's disease. Vitamin E has been shown to prevent free radical damage and delay memory deficits in animal studies. In a two-year study of people with Alzheimer's disease, large doses of vitamin E slowed progression of the disease. That said, when taken by healthy people, large doses of vitamin E have not been shown to *prevent* Alzheimer's disease. Vitamin E is considered nontoxic, even over the recommended dietary allowance (RDA) levels. The UL (upper limit) for vitamin E is set at 1,000 milligrams per day for adults over eighteen.

Foods rich in vitamin E include vegetable oils, nuts and seeds, wheat germ oil, peanut butter, and green leafy vegetables.

GO WITH THE FLOW

The psychologist Mihaly Csikszentmihalyi and a team of researchers at the University of Chicago were the first to describe and name the concept of flow, that state of concentration people get into when they feel fully involved in what they're doing. In the flow state, people become less self-aware and less distracted by outside concerns like what time it is or how hungry they are. People describe it as "losing yourself in the process" or "being in the zone." Experiencing flow is an excellent way to de-stress your brain.

Csikszentmihalyi's work identified intrinsic motivation as key to the flow experience. People who have intrinsic motivation can find the positives even in difficult situations, making them happier, more optimistic, and more creative than those who don't cultivate intrinsic motivation and who are only motivated by external rewards, like getting a paycheck. When you're in flow, your brain gets bathed in feel-good chemicals like dopamine and endorphins. Tasks that are too simple don't produce this state (because they cause boredom) and tasks that are too complex don't produce this state, either (because they cause stress and frustration). The task must be just right, requiring you to challenge your skills. You also need to care about what you're doing. If you think the task is pointless, then even if it stretches your skills you're unlikely to find flow. One way to add flow to your life is to add complexity to simple tasks, like trying to do them quickly. Another is to add purpose to tasks, such as thinking about how much more relaxing your house will feel if it's not so cluttered. Finally, you can seek out activities known to produce flow, such as hiking, painting, and writing.

QUIT SMOKING

You know smoking hurts your heart and your lungs. Before you light up again, consider the risk to your brain. Recent research shows that smokers have a thinner cerebral cortex, the area of the brain responsible for thinking, memory, perception, and language. If you quit smoking, some of the damage can be reversed—although it's better not to have smoked at all. Smoking also constricts blood flow to your brain and makes your blood more prone to clotting, increasing your risk of stroke. In addition, nicotine damages the interior walls of blood vessels and makes them more susceptible to atherosclerosis (hardening of the arteries). That also increases the chance of stroke. The good news? Your body starts repairing the damage within days of that last cigarette. If you quit smoking now, you reduce your risk for dementia and other forms of cognitive decline.

STOP STROKES

Stroke, the destruction of brain cells that occurs when blood to the brain is cut off, can kill you (it's the fifth leading cause of death in the US). If it doesn't kill you, it may leave you physically and/or mentally impaired—permanently. Stroke can be caused by blood clots or hardening of the arteries (atherosclerosis), although occasionally it is the result of trauma. Your chance of a stroke increases dramatically after you hit fifty-five and continues increasing as you age. Current research from a long-term study on Alzheimer's and aging suggests that having a stroke can put you at greater risk for developing Alzheimer's.

Risk factors for stroke include:

1. High blood pressure
2. Heart disease
3. Smoking
4. High cholesterol
5. Diabetes

If you have any of these risk factors, take concrete steps to safeguard your brain.

BE HAPPY

You remember that old saying, "Let a smile be your umbrella"? Well, we're not suggesting you give up your rain gear. But being optimistic—that is, feeling generally positive and confident about the future and about succeeding at various goals you may have—has protective powers. Recent studies show a correlation between being optimistic and reduced anxiety. Optimistic people were shown to have a larger orbitofrontal cortex (OFC). The OFC is known to help regulate emotion. In fact, if you experience a traumatic event (and presumably get a ding to your optimism), your OFC loses heft. Chronic stress reduces the ability of brain cells to connect to the OFC and instead helps produce pathways to anxiety (thanks, stress). Researchers theorize that just as stress and trauma can reduce the OFC, optimism and positive thinking may be able to build it back up again.

Other studies show a connection between higher levels of optimism and lower levels of the stress hormone cortisol. Being happy-go-lucky is better for your brain!

The truth is, realistic people are more accurate about how the world actually works, but optimistic people protect their brains. So, choose optimism when you can. How? Here are a few simple suggestions:

- Keep busy—dwelling on problems makes you less optimistic.
- Use affirmations—doggone it, people like you!
- Acknowledge success—it's easy to overlook when things go well.
- Use fewer negative words—stop yourself when you say "can't" and "never."
- Seek help dealing with your past—put painful experiences behind you.

AVOID ALZHEIMER'S

Alzheimer's disease, a devastating type of dementia that causes problems with memory, thinking, and behavior, has two types: early-onset (sometimes called younger-onset) and late-onset. Late-onset Alzheimer's is the culprit in most cases of lost mental function in people over sixty-five. Early-onset is much rarer. Only about 5 percent of those who develop Alzheimer's show signs of it before age sixty-five. The brains of Alzheimer's patients contain distinctive, abnormally shaped proteins known as tangles and plaques. Tangles are found inside neurons while plaques typically form outside the neurons in adjacent brain tissue. Tangles and plaques most commonly afflict the brain areas related to memory. In the 1980s, researchers found that a compound in plaques known as amyloid protein may actually be poisonous to brain cells. More recent research suggests that a protein called tau may be responsible for the telltale tangles found in the brains of Alzheimer's patients. In healthy brains tau proteins give neurons structural support, but in Alzheimer's patients this structural support collapses into useless twists and tangles.

To minimize your risk for Alzheimer's, change your lifestyle to a healthy one: good diet, lots of exercise, and plenty of mental stimulation.

HAVE SOME COFFEE

Your morning cup of coffee used to get a bad rap. All that caffeine! What were you thinking? But these days coffee has undergone a bit of rehab. Researchers have found it's not such a shady character. In fact, drinking a cup of coffee every morning can benefit your brain. Coffee does two things to help you:

1. First, it reduces the production of the neurotransmitter adenosine by binding to its receptors. Adenosine is a chemical that makes you feel tired. So you want adenosine at bedtime, but not when you have to go in there and ask the boss for a raise. Drinking a cup of coffee will make you feel more alert and focused.

2. Second, caffeine keeps your brain from reabsorbing dopamine, a feel-good neurotransmitter. That means you feel happy for longer.

One study showed that drinking coffee reduced depression among subjects—and even reduced suicidal tendencies. Some evidence also shows that coffee-drinking may help protect against Parkinson's and Alzheimer's.

But of course you can have too much of a good thing. Once you go over about 400 milligrams of caffeine per day—about four cups of coffee—the downside starts to outweigh the upside. For example, too much caffeine can give you migraines. It can cause insomnia, restlessness, and (because it's a diuretic) increased urination. Also, drinking coffee on an empty stomach can cause heartburn. For some people, coffee makes them jittery and nervous. This is especially true for individuals who already have anxiety. If you experience any of these side effects, reduce your consumption.

COUNT YOUR BREATHS

You know how you're always supposed to count to ten when you get angry? That's because giving yourself a little space before reacting can calm you down. Instead of the original outburst you were going to make, you're able to respond more calmly. The same idea holds true for counting your breaths. When you're upset, anxious, or worried, take a moment to focus on your breath. Don't worry about trying to control your breathing, just take a few deep breaths, then start counting: inhale + exhale = one breath. In a few moments you won't be so stressed. This is because counting your breaths is a kind of mindfulness—you're keeping your focus on the present and not thinking about anything else that's happening. And mindfulness, as we know from many studies, is a practice that can help improve memory and build cognitive skills. No special mantra or meditation is needed. Just count to ten!

COMBAT DEPRESSION

Depression, which is a mood disorder that involves feeling sad and uninterested, affects many people. For some people, an episode of depression might be mild—it might be, for example, related to a loss from which they gradually recover. For others, depression is so deep and long-lasting that even simple things like getting out of bed to shower become a monumental struggle. Of course it is bad for your brain to be mired in depression. If you feel depressed, especially if the feeling goes on for many days and keeps you from your normal activities, getting professional help is your first step. In addition to seeking help, there are things you can do to help combat depression:

1. Create structure. Give yourself a schedule, such as getting out of bed at a certain time, even if you don't feel like it, and eating on a regular timetable. Daily goals, like showering and getting dressed every day, are very helpful for combating depression.
2. Go for a walk. Getting a little exercise even just a few times a week can help your brain produce the feel-good chemicals that will give you a lift.
3. Eat right. You need good nutrition now more than ever.
4. Make a change. Do something different. Take a class, join a club, think new thoughts.
5. Get your shut-eye—but not too much. Most people need seven to nine hours of sleep per night to function well. Depressed people often sleep more or less than this. Do your best to get the right amount of sleep.
6. Do things you used to find fun, enjoyable, or rewarding. Even if you don't find them that much fun now, do them anyway. You just have to keep trying.

JOURNAL IT

Keeping a daily journal—by hand, not on your laptop—benefits your brain. Recent studies show that writing by hand enhances your memory, helps both sides of your brain coordinate (integrating information from both sides of your brain helps you improve your perception), and inspires thought and creativity because the slower process allows for reflection. You also use more of your brain, specifically the motor cortex, when you write instead of type. A stimulated brain is a healthy brain! Writing by hand also helps relieve stress, as repetitive actions can have a calming effect. This is particularly true if you write something calming, like five things you feel grateful for rather than all the ways you hate your boss.

STOP MULTITASKING

Trying to do a lot of things at once is supposed to be a sign that you're smart and productive. But new research shows that multitasking—doing more than one task at a time—has very big drawbacks. First, your brain can't actually multitask. What it does is switch from one task to the other, back and forth, back and forth. The problem? Your brain doesn't perform as well when it is constantly distracted this way. It's likely that the quality and efficiency of your work will suffer. For the vast majority of people, it's actually quicker for them to do tasks sequentially—plus they're less likely to make mistakes. A small percentage of people are actually good multitaskers—their brains are capable of handling more than one task at a time—but you'd be wise not to count yourself among them. In fact, one study showed that people who thought they were good at multitasking were actually the worst at it. Another study showed that people trying to deal with several tasks at once had significantly more problems paying attention and remembering information than those who did one task at a time. Habitual multitaskers actually train their brains to be less efficient. They have trouble organizing thoughts and focusing on what is important. As a consequence, they end up being slower, cumulatively, than those who do one thing at a time. Give your brain a break by giving up your multitasking ways!

SIP SOME GREEN TEA

Folklore says green tea helps you achieve deeper states of consciousness, especially during meditation. Science says green tea contains an amino acid called theanine, which aids in increasing concentration and attention while reducing fatigue and stress.

The most popular and potent version of green tea is called matcha. To create matcha, the plant is shaded from the sun for about three weeks before harvest. Shading the plant increases the levels of theanine. The ground powder made from these shaded green tea leaves is mixed directly into hot water to create the drink. (Tea is usually made by infusion, where the leaves are strained from the drink.) Drinking a mixture rather than an infusion allows your body to absorb more nutrients.

Green tea contains antioxidants and nutrients that improve your brain's performance. Green tea also contains polyphenols, which may improve memory, learning, and cognitive function.

LEND A HAND

You know that volunteering is good for your community. Did you know it's also good for your brain? Researchers have known for a long time that helping out others makes you feel better. Your brain produces dopamine and endorphins and other feel-good chemicals when you reach out to help. But a recent study conducted by Johns Hopkins Bloomberg School of Public Health showed even longer-lasting benefits than that momentary glow of goodness. The study found that people who volunteered maintained or increased the size of their memory centers (which usually decrease over time). Volunteering also helped women in particular improve their physical health, which of course is crucial to brain health. Researchers theorize that these physical improvements could help improve executive function (decision making). Another study showed that volunteers have lower blood pressure, which means less likelihood of stroke and other health problems.

Key elements of brain-boosting volunteering include working in teams (socializing helps the brain), problem-solving (practice makes perfect), and sharing knowledge (having a purpose makes your brain happy). In other words, simple tasks you perform by yourself are unlikely to boost your brain as much.

TOMATO IT UP

Your brain loves carotenoids, which, among other things, help chase away free radicals before they can do too much damage. And tomatoes have lots of carotenoids, so eat up! In recent research, people with cognitive problems and those with Alzheimer's all showed higher levels of carotenoids in their blood after eating tomatoes. When you cook down tomatoes, you actually make it easier for your body to absorb the carotenoids, so ladle on the marinara. Since carotenoids are fat-soluble, a little olive oil in the sauce helps your body absorb even more of these do-good chemicals. But don't skin them! That's where much of the nutrition hangs out.

FAST-TRACK YOUR METABOLISM

Everything your body does, from warding off infection to digesting your dinner to sending blood to your brain, occurs through a process called metabolism. During metabolism, cells break down chemicals and nutrients to generate energy and form new molecules, like proteins. Metabolism in brain cells affects how information is signaled, according to a recent study by McGill University and University of Zurich researchers. Researchers concluded that this is why a special diet can help some individuals with seizure disorder control their seizures. In other words, there is a link between how brain cells create energy and how they communicate. Brain glucose metabolism also affects brain function, particularly memory. Research shows that maintaining stable glucose concentrations in your brain is healthier for your brain, and that levels that are too high or low have a negative effect on brain function.

To fast-track your metabolism:

- Start off your day with breakfast. This wakes up your metabolism.
- Graze with small meals and snacks throughout the day to maintain a more stable metabolism. Avoid the peaks and valleys associated with eating large meals less frequently.
- Eat enough—but not too much. Undereating and overeating both damage your metabolism.
- Skip artificial sweeteners. These may interfere with your body's metabolism.
- Sip a cuppa. A cup of coffee helps boost metabolism.

TRY THE OTHER HAND

If you're like most people in the world, you have a dominant hand—one hand that handles most tasks. Call it your go-to hand. If we had to guess, we'd say you're right-handed (about 90 percent of people are). Only a tiny percentage—about 1 percent—of people use both hands equally (this is referred to as being ambidextrous). This is because your brain is lazy. For one-handed tasks, such as writing a note, it defaults to same-old, same-old. One way to ward off cognitive decline is to get out of this rut. You need to stimulate your brain—make it do something in a new way. Since the left side of your brain controls the motor function on the right side of your body (and vice versa), by switching which hand you do a task with, you'll light up a different part of your brain. For example, brush your teeth with your nondominant hand. Put your fork in your nondominant hand and eat your dinner that way (bonus points for not spilling all over your shirt). The fact that these tasks likely feel awkward is a sign that you're engaging your brain in a new way.

WALK IT OFF

Any exercise is good for your brain, but walking in particular has some significant benefits. Researchers at New Mexico Highlands University found that "the foot's impact during walking sends pressure waves through the arteries that significantly modify and can increase the supply of blood to the brain" (ScienceDaily.com).

Furthermore, walking elevates your mood, which is good. And when you're wrestling with a knotty problem, a long walk can stimulate the creative centers of your brain, helping you to figure out a resolution. There's also evidence that walking improves your memory skills. So put on those walking shoes and get started.

BECOME ANTI-SOCIAL (MEDIA)

For all the good that connecting with old friends on social media can create, it can also do bad things for your brain. You've probably had that experience where you go to check *Facebook* for just a few minutes and three hours later wonder what happened to the time. (Look at the kitties!) Or you anxiously await your friends' "Likes" and ponder when you turned into a lab rat pressing the lever for pellets. A German study showed that one in three people say they feel worse after spending time on *Facebook* than they did before, with "worse" meaning lonely, frustrated, and/or sad. Another study showed that the more people used *Facebook*, the worse they felt. Researchers call this "*Facebook* depression." So much for the joy of connecting with friends. And that thing about the lab rat? It's true: being on social media can feed your brain's tendency toward addiction. It wants rewards, and what's more rewarding than seeing a thumbs-up on your post? One study at Stanford University showed that people who spent a lot of time on social media have trouble filtering out unimportant information and have more trouble remembering things. But that doesn't mean you have to quit social media cold turkey and go live in a cabin in the woods. In moderation, connecting with others via social media can help you stay informed, help you express yourself, and help you become part of a greater community. The key word is *moderation*.

GET HIGH ON ENDORPHINS

Did you know that exercise has been shown to help combat major depression? It's true. Exercise produces feel-good chemicals, such as endorphins, that help boost mood. Endorphins are neurotransmitters, which are chemicals that help your nerve cells send signals. Endorphins protect you from feeling pain and help elevate your mood. Exercise isn't the only way to prompt your brain to reward you with those beneficial chemicals, though. You can also stimulate their production by smelling certain aromas, like lavender. Or you can eat something spicy. The burning sensation, caused by capsaicin, prompts the brain to release endorphins. Not a fan of spice? Any of your favorite foods can help move your happiness needle up a notch.

RAW IS FOR RABBITS

Although raw food proponents claim that when you cook food you destroy its nutritional value, research shows that sometimes the opposite is true. Several studies show that cooking food actually helps people access the nutrition in it. For example, one carotenoid, lycopene, is hard for the body to absorb from uncooked food. One study showed that people who ate raw diets had low levels of lycopene. Cooking also allows other antioxidants to become more freely available. Carotenoids and antioxidants are essential to brain health.

However, it is true that some vitamins are lost during the cooking process, such as vitamin C and some B vitamins. But overall, cooking improves the bioavailability of nutrients. By occasionally eating raw food you can balance the nutrition you're getting. Steaming and boiling are the healthiest choices, although if roasting is what it takes to get you to eat your veggies, then do it!

PUMP IRON

Your brain needs iron. Iron helps with cognitive functions—for example, children who have an iron deficiency tend to do worse on math and language tests. Recent studies show that even minor levels of iron deficiency can have negative effects on brain function. Iron is necessary for the production of myelin, the insulating sheath around neurons (nerve cells), which helps speed the rate at which cells convey impulses. Without appropriate myelination, the nervous system, including your brain, cannot function correctly. If you have an iron deficiency, you may need to rely on supplementation rather than diet to raise your iron content to normal levels. But don't overdo it. Taking iron supplements can cause side effects such as nausea, vomiting, constipation, diarrhea, dark-colored stools, and/or abdominal distress. To minimize these side effects, follow your doctor's recommendations and take with food.

TRY THE SPICY LIFE

Turmeric (*Curcuma longa*), sometimes called curcumin, is a common ingredient in curry powder and has been used for centuries in traditional medicine mostly for its pain-relieving and anti-inflammatory properties. Researchers became interested in the brain-protecting properties of the herb because people in India, who tend to eat a lot of curry and thus turmeric, have lower rates of Alzheimer's than people in other countries who don't eat the spice or who don't eat as much of it.

One recent study showed that turmeric may help the brain repair itself and grow new cells, which could help in the treatment of neurological disorders like Alzheimer's and Parkinson's. Another study showed that the anti-inflammatory properties of turmeric may help heal brain damage in Alzheimer's patients. An analysis of various studies of turmeric shows that it may help lower cholesterol (and therefore may help lessen the chance of stroke) and that it may prevent neurotoxicity by binding to metals like iron and copper. However, most curcumin is eliminated from the body rather than being used by it, so absorption is a problem. It should be taken with food. If you have liver or gall bladder problems, you should avoid turmeric, especially heavy doses that occur with supplementation. It may interact with blood thinners and NSAIDs, so check with your healthcare provider if you take those types of drugs. Otherwise, now's the time to learn to love curry!

LAUGH!

That's right: laugh! It really is the best medicine—for both our minds and our bodies. For one thing, a good sense of humor provides needed stress relief. When we laugh at our problems rather than fret over them, they can feel less serious and thus seem easier to solve. Humor also improves cognitive function by keeping the mind active and encouraging creative thinking—a vital defense against age-related impairments—and it provides an important emotional catharsis during periods of emotional tension. Laughing also benefits the heart, improves oxygen flow to the brain, lowers your blood pressure, and works the muscles in the head, neck, chest, and pelvis—in much the same way as the stress-reduction exercises of yoga. This helps keep muscles loose and limber and enables them to rest more easily. When you laugh, your body activates T cells, which help you fight off disease. So rent a funny movie, go to a comedy club, or watch a comedy show and laugh!

CHANGE YOUR JOB

At any given time, as many as 40 percent of workers hate their jobs. You may think that's the trade-off you make for being able to pay the mortgage—but hating your job is bad for your brain. Although we tend to think that jobs are supposed to suck, people who enjoy their work overall tend to be more productive and successful. An Ohio State University study showed that people who felt unsatisfied in their jobs had higher levels of depression and insomnia. They also worried more than people who enjoyed their jobs.

Something else to think about: how stimulating your job is. Jobs that require little mental engagement or which require a lot of alone time tend to be worse for your brain. A report by the University of Wisconsin showed that jobs that require complex social interaction actually help prevent Alzheimer's. Jobs that require thinking on your feet also help protect the brain. So, take a good look at your job. Is it helping or hurting your brain?

GET MOVING

Regular physical exercise keeps you mentally strong. Researchers recommend clocking at least twenty minutes a day, but thirty minutes to one hour daily is better. Aerobic exercise such as running or swimming helps get the blood coursing through your system, carrying oxygen and glucose to your brain—two substances your brain can't do without. Regular exercise also can prod the brain to make more molecules that help protect and produce neurons. Though studies are still underway to establish the link between exercise and increased brain neurons, many researchers—including those involved with Alzheimer's disease research—are studying the protective effects of regular physical exercise on the brain's neural paths for transmitting signals. According to the US Office of Disease Prevention and Health Promotion, physical activity guidelines suggest that 150 minutes of moderate-intensity aerobic activity per week can lower the risk of premature death, coronary heart disease, stroke, hypertension, type 2 diabetes, and depression.

Beyond the physical benefits, exercise offers emotional benefits. It increases self-esteem and confidence, which makes you stand up straighter and look the rest of the world squarely in the eye.

LIFT A LOAD

Don't stick to just one type of exercise, like aerobics, to build your brain cells. A 2016 study showed a correlation between weight training and dramatically improved cognitive function in a group of older adults suffering cognitive decline. Stretching exercises alone didn't help. Most health specialists say thirty to forty minutes of weight training a week is sufficient to maintain optimum health. Weight training can vastly improve muscle strength, balance, and flexibility—all of which are good for your brain.

DON'T OVERDO IT

A study of male Harvard graduates compared longevity rates of major athletes (meaning those who lettered in a particular sport), minor athletes (those who participated but didn't letter), and nonathletes. It was assumed that the major athletes, who presumably exercised the hardest, would have the greatest longevity, but, in fact, it was the minor athletes who lived the longest.

What does this mean? Well, for starters, when it comes to life-extending physical activity, moderation is best. There's no need to train like an Olympic athlete, because too much exercise is just as bad as too little. Studies suggest that overexercising actually decreases the number of new brain cells your body creates. In one study, rats that overexercised produced half as many brain cells as rats who hadn't even exercised at all. Of course rats aren't people, but researchers theorize a correlation to human overexercising.

The key is to strengthen and maintain your body's and brain's systems, not abuse them, which is what an excessive physical regimen does. If you feel pain, you may be working too hard. Slow down and listen to your body. It will tell you what it needs and when you've gone too far.

FOCUS ON BETTER, NOT BEST

A study shows that eating exactly seven walnuts a day boosts your brain power. Researchers show that spending at least sixty-eight minutes a day doing aerobic exercise is best for your brain. The list goes on. The number of best practices for your brain is long—and a little daunting. Learning how to pick the "better" option instead of struggling to attain the "best" one can help. Trying to achieve perfection is the enemy of making progress. Sure, maybe ninety minutes of aerobics a day is ideal, but a brisk thirty-minute walk every afternoon is much better than remaining glued to the sofa. Think of it this way: there's a poor choice, a better choice, and a best choice. You want to avoid the poor choices, pick as many best choices as you can, and for the rest, go with "better." It's better for your brain health if you make some good choices rather than none—or give up because it seems too hard. For example, you know that the saturated fats in cheese make it food to avoid. But if you love cheese and can't imagine living without it, pick an aged Cheddar. That's much better for you than a processed slice of goop. When making choices, ask yourself "What's better?"

WALK AND TALK

One of the best ways to strengthen your brain is to exercise it physically and mentally—at the same time. Exercising your brain by thinking—working out problems—is beneficial. And exercising your brain by taking it for a walk is also good. The hippocampus, the part of the brain concerned with memory, grows as your body gets fitter. But now German scientists have shown that if you do both at the same time, you reap even greater benefits. For example, if you bicycle or walk while learning a new language, the vocabulary tends to stick in your memory longer. Note that this is not the same as multitasking, where you're trying to do two mental activities at once, like reading a book while listening to a lecture. It's the combination of physical and mental activity that is key.

GET GOTU KOLA

Don't mistake this herb for the caffeine-containing kola nut. Gotu kola (*Centella asiatica*), also known as Indian or Asian pennywort, contains no caffeine. It is in the same plant family as carrots and parsnips. Because it helps rebuild energy reserves, it has become known as "food for the brain." In traditional medicine, it's used to increase mental and physical strength, combat stress, and improve reflexes. Recent studies have shown that it improves circulation by increasing the flow of blood throughout the body and strengthening veins and capillaries. A pharmacological review of its component chemicals suggests there is some scientific basis for claims that it has antidepressive properties and can help improve concentration and attention span. It is typically taken as an extract or in capsule form; follow the label's directions. Pregnant women should not use this herb, nor should anyone with an overactive thyroid condition.

TAKE MARVELOUS MELATONIN

Melatonin, which you may know as the sleep hormone, can help protect your brain. Some research indicates that melatonin can help keep brain cells from dying, which is good news for people with strokes, Alzheimer's, and other brain-cell-destroying diseases. Melatonin is an antioxidant (it sucks up those nasty free radicals) and can help calm inflammation of neurons, which can help keep your brain healthy. And, of course, your body produces melatonin to help you sleep, which is good for your brain. For many years, people have taken melatonin supplements to help them fight insomnia.

One study suggests that melatonin may help reduce brain swelling in cases of traumatic brain injury, although the evidence is preliminary. It is also being studied as a potential treatment for injuries to the central nervous system, such as spinal cord injuries. A different study suggests that melatonin can help protect brains in people with Parkinson's. It can also help reduce the effects of sleep deprivation.

Melatonin passes the blood-brain barrier, so if you eat it, it will go to work in your brain (this isn't true of all the good-for-your-brain chemicals researchers know about). You can get melatonin from your diet by eating these foods:

- Almonds
- Fenugreek (spice)
- Goji berries
- Mustard seeds
- Orange bell peppers
- Raspberries
- Tomatoes
- Walnuts

You can also take a melatonin supplement, although obviously it is better to take it at bedtime versus first thing in the morning.

REACH FOR RIBOFLAVIN

Riboflavin, also known as vitamin B_2, plays a key role in releasing energy from macronutrients to all cells of the body. It also helps change the amino acid tryptophan into niacin, another B vitamin. Riboflavin contributes to normal growth, production of certain hormones, formation of red blood cells, and nerve function. The metabolic function of B vitamins (releasing energy from micronutrients) is particularly crucial to brain health.

The recommended dietary allowance (RDA) for vitamin B_2 is 1.6 milligrams for men aged twenty-three to fifty, 1.4 milligrams for men fifty-one and older, 1.3 milligrams for women up to age twenty-two, and 1.2 milligrams for women twenty-three and older. Pregnant women require an additional 0.3 milligrams daily, and women who are breastfeeding require an extra 0.5 milligrams. Riboflavin has no established UL (upper limit), but moderation is always best.

Foods rich in riboflavin include:

- Beef liver
- Enriched-grain foods
- Green leafy vegetables
- Low-fat yogurt
- Milk
- Whole-grain foods

PILE ON THE ONIONS

It may not do any favors for your dating life, but piling on the onions can help protect your brain. A recent study showed that certain chemical compounds found in onions may help protect the brain from stroke damage. Onions are known to contain antioxidants that can remove free radicals (which are especially hard on your brain). Onions also have polyphenols, which are linked to improved cerebral blood flow and metabolism, and other flavonoids that help protect the brain against toxins. And onions are full of vitamin C, vitamin B_6, and folate, nutrients that help protect your brain. So, apologize to your date and crunch an onion.

ADD SOME A

Vitamin A, an antioxidant, helps protect brain cells from harmful free radicals and benefits the circulatory system so blood flow to the brain remains strong. Vitamin A is essential to memory and learning. It also promotes healthy cells and tissues.

Vitamin A comes in several forms. Retinol, known as preformed vitamin A, is found in animal foods. Another form of vitamin A is a group called carotenoids, which includes beta-carotene. Beta-carotene is the carotenoid most readily converted by the body into vitamin A.

Foods rich in vitamin A (retinol) include beef liver, fish oil, and fortified foods such as milk. Foods rich in vitamin A (beta-carotene) include sweet potatoes, carrots, kale, spinach, apricots, cantaloupe, broccoli, and winter squash.

Most supplements break down vitamin A into beta-carotene and retinol on their labels. Too much retinol can lead to headaches, dry and scaly skin, bone and joint pain, liver damage, vomiting, loss of appetite, abnormal bone growth, nerve damage, and birth defects. Even though beta-carotene is not toxic to the body, it's better not to overdo it. Vitamin A has a UL (upper limit) set at 3,000 micrograms (mcg) or 10,000 IU (international units) per day for adults over eighteen.

IT'S GR-APE!

A preliminary study in the *Journal of Neuroscience* found that grape seed extract may help prevent plaque formation in the brain, which is associated with Alzheimer's. There is also some evidence that it can protect against brain injury in the case of stroke, both before and after a stroke event, and that it may protect against neurotoxins. Grape seed extract contains antioxidants, which help prevent free radicals from damaging brain cells. It also has other brain-protecting compounds and can cross the blood-brain barrier. Taken as a supplement, it is generally believed to be safe but should be avoided by children, pregnant women and nursing mothers, and people who are allergic to grapes. Consult with your healthcare provider if you're taking other drugs or have high blood pressure or a bleeding disorder. Side effects may include headache or nausea.

PACK IN THE PROTEIN

Protein supplies the amino acids your brain needs to produce neurotransmitters such as serotonin, which helps regulate moods. Put simply, you need protein for happiness.

However, when it comes to protein, your body uses only what it needs and stores the extra as body fat. Eating large amounts of protein, especially from animal foods, can increase your saturated fat (bad fat) and cholesterol intake. It can also cause you to crowd out other important foods, such as grains, fruits, and vegetables, creating a nutritional imbalance.

When your body digests protein, it produces toxic by-products. The kidneys filter these toxins out. So eating too much protein strains your kidneys. Also, consumption of excess protein requires more water to excrete urea, a waste product formed when protein turns to body fat. This increases the chances for dehydration and increases the need to urinate.

Athletes need only slightly more protein than the recommended dietary allowance (RDA). Generally, nonathletes need around ½ gram per pound of body weight, and most athletes need ½ to ¾ gram of protein per pound of body weight.

Keep in mind the following protein contents of common foods:

- A 3- to 4-ounce serving of lean meat, poultry, or fish contains about 25 to 35 grams of protein
- 1 cup of cooked beans or lentils contains about 18 grams of protein
- 1 cup of low-fat or fat-free milk contains 8 grams of protein
- 1 cup of low-fat yogurt contains about 10 grams of protein
- 1 cup of low-fat cottage cheese contains about 28 grams of protein
- 2 tablespoons of peanut butter contain about 7 grams of protein
- 2 ounces of low-fat cheese contain 14 to 16 grams of protein
- 1 serving of vegetables contains 1 to 3 grams of protein
- 1 serving of grain foods generally contains 3 to 6 grams of protein

SAFETY FIRST

The best way to protect your brain from injury is to avoid injury in the first place. If it doesn't kill you, traumatic brain injury can cause memory problems, thinking problems, seizures, paralysis, and more, both short and long term. Think about the tasks you perform each day and resolve to do them in a way that protects your brain. For example, when you're driving, wear your seatbelt and drive defensively. Sure, you may be justified in your road rage, but an accident (or a confrontation) can be bad for your brain! At home, use handrails, take your time going up and down steps, use an actual ladder instead of a chair. Falls and auto accidents are the two most common causes of traumatic brain injury (TBI), according to the Centers for Disease Control and Prevention. Striking or being struck (hitting an object or being hit by it, such as when playing sports) and physical violence (such as assault) are the next most common. Sometimes the cause isn't known or is the result of less-common situations, such as warfare (where a firearms attack or bomb blast can cause TBI). Put your safety first and protect your brain.

BOOST YOUR B$_{12}$

An estimated 25 percent of people between ages sixty and seventy are deficient in B$_{12}$, an essential nutrient. So are nearly 40 percent of people eighty and older. A B$_{12}$ deficiency may be mistaken for an age-related decline in mental function, including memory loss and a reduction in reasoning skills, and may affect mood.

Some potential benefits of B$_{12}$ supplements include the treatment of Alzheimer's disease and dementia, sleep disorders, and diabetic neuropathy. It is important to know that a deficiency of this vitamin can be hidden, and even progress, if extra folic acid is taken to treat or prevent anemia. There are no known toxic effects of taking large doses of vitamin B$_{12}$, but neither is there any scientific evidence that extra vitamin B$_{12}$ brings extra benefits. Vitamin B$_{12}$ has no established UL (upper limit). To hedge your bets, take a multivitamin tablet daily.

KEEP IT COOL

Heat injury, also called hyperthermia, happens when your body overheats. Often this occurs when people work hard outdoors during hot weather, but it can also occur just by being exposed to excessive heat or by being stuck indoors in a room with poor ventilation. In such situations, a range of heat injuries can occur, with heatstroke (a body temperature of 104°F or more) being the most damaging. Heatstroke is a medical emergency and the damage to your brain (and other organs) can be permanent. The damages to the brain can include problems with cognition, memory, and focus. Longer periods of exposure mean worse outcomes, so if you experience symptoms of heat injury, such as rapid breathing, nausea, headache, muscle cramps, or altered mental state, take shelter immediately and call 911. Cool down with a cool bath, ice packs, or the garden hose.

These situations contribute to the likelihood of heat injury:

- Wearing too much clothing for the conditions.
- Working in areas with elevated temperature, such as around ovens.
- Not getting enough sleep.
- Using alcohol or illegal drugs, such as meth or heroin.
- Not drinking enough water.
- Traveling or moving to a hot place from a cool one.
- Being old or young.
- Taking certain medications (check with your healthcare provider).
- Having certain medical problems, like circulatory problems, and heart, lung, or kidney diseases.
- Being very overweight or underweight.
- Having had heatstroke before.

Avoid overexertion during hot weather, drink plenty of water, take frequent breaks when outdoors, and spend time in air-conditioned places.

BREAK OUT THE B$_6$

Also known as pyridoxine and pyridoxal, vitamin B$_6$ helps the brain work properly, enables the body to resist stress, helps maintain the proper chemical balance in the body's fluids, works with other vitamins and minerals to supply the energy used by muscles, and is influential in cell growth. Like other B vitamins, B$_6$ helps convert sugar into glucose, which the brain needs for fuel. It also benefits general circulation, which can improve memory. Older people need substantially more B$_6$ than younger people, so the older you get, the more you'll want to add to your diet.

Vitamin B$_6$, in conjunction with folate (another B vitamin) and vitamin B$_{12}$, helps to lower blood levels of homocysteine, a risk factor for heart disease. The recommended dietary allowance (RDA) for vitamin B$_6$ is 2.2 milligrams for men and 2.0 milligrams for women. Pregnant women need an additional 0.6 milligrams each day, and breastfeeding women need an extra 0.5 milligrams daily. Don't exceed 100 milligrams a day without checking with your doctor; an excess of B$_6$ can be toxic.

Foods rich in B$_6$ include:

- Avocados
- Bananas
- Beef
- Carrots
- Chicken
- Fish
- Lentils
- Liver
- Rice
- Soybeans
- Whole grains

LET SOMEONE NEEDLE YOU

Acupuncture, a form of treatment in traditional Chinese medicine, is the process of inserting slender needles slightly under the skin at various points of the body in order to balance the flow of energy (chi) throughout the body. Traditionally, chi was believed to be blocked in ill people and acupuncture helped get it moving again. Whether you believe in the literal existence of chi or not, acupuncture can nonetheless help keep your brain healthy. Researchers have found that acupuncture can benefit people who are experiencing depression, anxiety, and other brain problems, including insomnia. Some researchers believe that your brain releases feel-good neurotransmitters in reaction to the needles, although there isn't complete agreement on how acupuncture works. One study showed that people treated with acupuncture had less anxiety and a better memory afterward, as compared to a control group that didn't undergo acupuncture. For mood disorders, acupuncture can work immediately, unlike prescription drugs or talk therapy. It has few side effects (except for that pesky needles-hurt-going-in part). Acupuncture also shows promise as an aid for alcohol- and other drug-dependency issues, although research into this area is preliminary and ongoing.

Acupuncture is one of those treatments where the adage "Don't try this at home!" applies. Instead, seek out a licensed acupuncturist (licensing varies from state to state).

A related practice, acupressure, uses firm touch rather than needles to stimulate the flow of chi throughout the body. It has not been studied as much as acupuncture, but it can be a good place to start if you don't like the idea of people poking needles into you.

THIS IS YOUR BRAIN...

...this is your brain on drugs. Now don't roll your eyes. We know you've heard this before, but it bears repeating. Use of illicit drugs like heroin, cocaine, and methamphetamine is very hard on your brain. Not only do addiction and drug tolerance make you crave the drug in ever-increasing quantities, they create potential legal, social, and personal safety issues. But the worst risk is how long-term illicit drug use alters your brain. It impairs your cognition, making it harder for you to think. You will have a harder time making decisions, understanding situations, or knowing what to do. Your memory is affected and you will have more trouble controlling your behavior. And that's even when you're not taking the drug—you can't reverse this damage to your brain once it's done. And when you're under the influence, all of these problems are magnified. If you don't use illicit drugs now, don't start. If you do use these drugs, the good news is you can keep your brain problems from getting worse by getting help and quitting now.

AN APPLE A DAY...

Studies have shown that eating apples may help prevent stroke. The active ingredient in apple pulp is pectin, a soluble form of fiber that helps reduce "bad" cholesterol by keeping it in the intestinal tract until it is eliminated. European studies indicate that apple pectin can help to eliminate lead, mercury, and other toxic heavy metals from the human body (heavy metals are believed to affect cognition and behavior). Quercetin, a polyphenol found in apples, is believed to help repair damage from free radicals. And apples also help your brain produce the neurotransmitter acetylcholine, important to muscle control and for promoting REM sleep.

It's important to thoroughly wash apples and to avoid eating the seeds, which can be poisonous. Do eat the peel—that's where most of the nutrition resides. (But choose organic so you're not eating pesticides!) All apples provide nutrients, but eating a variety of apple types is the best way to ensure you're getting as many nutrients as possible.

SMILE A WHILE

It turns out that those people who are always advising you to smile are right—smiling makes you feel better and improves your mood. (The truth of this matter does not negate the fact that anyone who tells you to smile is an annoying jerk. We fully agree, although we know that since we just told you to smile, that means we're the annoying jerks...)

A Penn State study showed that people who smiled were perceived as more likable, more polite, and even more competent than those who did not. Other studies have shown that when you smile, you fool your brain into thinking you're happy. This is true even if your smile is fake. Your brain stops thinking so many Eeyore thoughts and you are more likely to perceive the positives in the world around you. One researcher suggests that smiling can even help protect your brain from stress. So put on a happy face!

GO BIG ON B$_1$

Vitamin B$_1$, also called thiamine, is a potent antioxidant—which you probably remember as the thing that fights damaging free radicals. Thiamine helps the body use carbohydrates effectively, so it's essential to metabolism—in fact, it is used to treat problems with metabolism. A serious deficiency in vitamin B$_1$ can even result in dementia! Brain problems associated with vitamin B$_1$ deficiency include confusion, memory loss, and mood changes such as apathy. Some evidence supports the belief that thiamine can help increase energy and improve learning. People who drink a lot of alcohol have a high risk of B$_1$ deficiency. The recommended dietary allowance (RDA) for adults is 1.1 milligrams per day for women and 1.2 milligrams per day for men. Researchers don't have enough information on adverse effects to set a UL (upper limit). You can find vitamin B$_1$ in yeast, meat, nuts, beans, and in cereal grains like oats and rice.

SOLVE REAL PUZZLES

For a while there everyone was doing crosswords to stave off Alzheimer's, but current research says they don't help with overall cognition or memory. They're fun, so feel free to continue, but to really boost your brain, you should solve real-world problems. For example, instead of just writing down your grocery list, create a mental picture of the grocery store and organize your list according to what aisle you'll start with and which you'll end with. Or you could alphabetize all the groceries or memorize the list or something similar. The point is to do something that wakes up your brain. The problem is that many of the activities we do throughout the day are repetitive—we drive to the same grocery store to buy the same foods to cook in the same recipes. So by engaging your brain more, you'll help boost cognition.

FILL UP ON FIBER

Fiber improves your digestion, reduces your risk of colon cancer, and can help you lose weight by making you feel full. And fiber contributes to brain health. Scientists in Great Britain found that for every 7 grams of fiber you include in your diet each day, your risk of a stroke goes down 7 percent. That's a pretty big benefit!

Unfortunately, many people don't consume enough fiber. Adding it to your diet may be easier than you think. Here are some tips that can help you get started:

- Look at the fiber content on the Nutrition Facts label on packaged foods. Good sources of fiber have at least 2.5 grams of fiber per serving.
- Substitute higher-fiber foods, such as whole-grain breads, brown rice, whole-wheat pasta, and fruits and vegetables, for lower-fiber foods such as white bread, white rice, candy, and chips.
- Eat more raw vegetables and fresh fruits, and include the skins when appropriate.
- Plan to eat high-fiber foods, such as fruits, vegetables, legumes, and whole-grain starches, at every meal.
- Start your day with a high-fiber breakfast cereal, such as bran cereal or oatmeal. Look for cereals that contain at least 5 grams of fiber per serving. Add fresh fruit for an extra fiber boost.
- Eat a variety of high-fiber foods to ensure you get a mix of both soluble and insoluble fiber—both types are important to your health.
- Use snacks to increase your fiber intake by eating high-fiber foods, such as dried fruits, popcorn, and whole-wheat crackers.
- Try to eat legumes, or dried beans, at least two to three times per week. Add them to salads, soups, casseroles, or spaghetti sauce.
- Eat whole fruits more often than juice. Most of the fiber in fruit is found in the skin and pulp, which are removed when juicing.

FIGHT INFLAMMATION

The way your immune system repels infection naturally causes inflammation. In fact, inflammation is a sign your immune system is working right; it repels pesky bacterial invaders. Inflammation is also a sign that your body is working to repair itself after an injury. But not all inflammation is a sign of good health and healing. Many researchers believe a type of unhelpful inflammation occurs in some chronic diseases, including diseases of the brain such as Alzheimer's, Parkinson's, and depression. In the case of chronic diseases, instead of occurring briefly to deal with a one-time event, inflammation itself is believed to be chronic. It creates a cycle of damaging health cells, with that damage triggering more inflammation and more damage to cells.

Many trials of drug interventions to calm chronic inflammation have proved disappointing. Researchers theorize that the later such interventions happen, the harder it is for them to succeed. Catching chronic inflammation early, before it does significant damage, seems key to protecting the brain. For example, one study showed that taking NSAIDs with late-stage Alzheimer's actually created greater cognitive decline, whereas taking NSAIDs before signs of serious cognitive decline occurred seemed to slow cognitive decline. Although researchers don't have a clear understanding of the role of chronic inflammation in such diseases, reducing chronic inflammation probably helps reduce the likelihood that you'll suffer these diseases. The same steps that help you keep your brain healthy also help protect you against chronic inflammation. These preventive measures include not smoking, not drinking excessively, eating lots of fruits and vegetables, and using healthy oils when you cook. In addition, the Mayo Clinic suggests that herbal supplementation with cat's claw, devil's claw, mangosteen, or milk thistle may have promise in reducing chronic inflammation.

NOTCH UP THE NIACIN

Niacin, also known as vitamin B_3, promotes brain health. Your brain uses niacin, along with other B vitamins, to break down carbohydrates into energy. Although rare, a niacin deficiency can cause memory loss, confusion, and depression. Niacin increases good cholesterol and decreases bad cholesterol and triglycerides, which helps prevent strokes. Niacin supplements are even used to treat some types of schizophrenia, and niacin is being studied as a potential treatment for Alzheimer's, although, so far, results have been mixed.

Dietary sources of vitamin B_3 include whole-grain foods, fortified cereal, lean meat, fish, poultry, peanuts, brewer's yeast, yogurt, and sunflower seeds.

The recommended dietary allowance (RDA) for niacin is 14 milligrams per day for women and 16 milligrams per day for men. Because it's water-soluble, your body will get rid of extra amounts. Even so, don't overdo it! Niacin has a UL (upper limit) set at 35 milligrams per day for adults over eighteen.

MORE IS BETTER

Once upon a time, people believed that you use only 10 percent of your brain, that when you were born you had all the brain cells you were ever going to have, and that some people are left-brained and some people are right-brained. (Do you still believe that one? Lots of people do. But it's not true.)

Our understanding of the brain is always changing. So it might be that some of the brain hacks we've noted in this book will someday prove to be untrue, or that new research might cast doubt on previous conclusions. What's a brain-centric person to do? The answer is that the more brain-supporting things you do, the better. That way, if it turns out that one brain hack isn't effective (maybe blueberries aren't the superfood we think they are), you'll still have benefited because you've also exercised, volunteered, and eaten your carotenoids. In other words, the more you do to help keep your brain healthy, the better.

DRINK KOLA, NOT COLA

The kola nut, found in tropical Africa, is high in caffeine. Made into a tea, kola nut can help improve cerebral circulation, potentially reducing the risk of stroke. It also boosts oxygenation in your body, including in your brain, which means it can improve cognitive function. Traditionally, kola nut has been used to treat headaches.

Although the kola nut was once used in some cola drinks (for flavor), giving those drinks their name, today's cola drinks are either high in sugar or high in artificial sweeteners and so don't pass the "Is it healthy for my brain?" test. Instead of drinking cold carbonated cola drinks, try an infusion (tea) of kola nut. Because of the caffeine, it will stimulate your brain, so think of it when you need to revive your flagging energy. It is also believed to block some neurotransmitters and boost others, like dopamine, so it can be used as a mood elevator. If you're not a fan of tea, you can also find kola nut as a liquid supplement, a capsule supplement, a syrup, a tincture, a gel, in a blend with other herbs for taste, in a new old-fashioned cola drink, or as an actual food product (be forewarned: the first bite can taste quite bitter!).

If you have high blood pressure, heart problems, or are sensitive to caffeine, then the kola nut in any of its forms is not for you. Otherwise, give it a try and see how well it clears your mind.

MINIMIZE MERCURY

Research shows that even low levels of mercury may contribute to Alzheimer's disease. Nerve cells exposed to mercury form the tangles and plaques often present in Alzheimer's cases. In an article published in the journal *NeuroReport Canadian* researcher Dr. Boyd Haley said, "Seven of the characteristic markers that we look for to distinguish Alzheimer's disease can be produced in normal brain tissues, or cultures of neurons, by the addition of extremely low levels of mercury."

Most people are exposed to mercury through eating fish, although mercury can also be found in pollution. Fish, although a lean source of protein, full of vitamins and minerals, and high in omega-3 fatty acids, may contain high levels of mercury. Fish contaminated with mercury should be avoided. In 2017 the FDA and EPA issued guidelines about eating fish for certain groups, such as women who are pregnant. According to the Mayo Clinic this advice is suitable for everyone to follow. The 2017 report categorizes fish into three groups: best choices, good choices, and choices to avoid (highest mercury levels):

- Best choices include catfish, haddock, salmon, shrimp, tilapia, and canned light tuna.
- Good choices include bluefish, grouper, halibut, and canned albacore/white tuna.
- Choices to avoid are king mackerel, marlin, orange roughy, shark, swordfish, tilefish (sourced from the Gulf of Mexico), and bigeye tuna.

TRY A NEW FOOD

Your brain is lazy. (Everyone's brain is lazy.) It wants to lie there like a lizard in the sun instead of actually working. That's one of the reasons why you make the same old meals week after week when you could try a new recipe every night for the rest of your life and still not get to the end of all the cookbooks on your shelf. To give your brain a kick in the pants, go ahead and try something new. If you eat a lot of Italian, make something Thai. You'll more fully engage your brain figuring out a new recipe, working with different ingredients, and learning new cooking skills and techniques. Plus, eating a variety of foods prepared in a variety of ways helps make sure your brain is getting the whole range of micronutrients it needs.

FEED YOURSELF FOLIC

Folic acid, also known as vitamin B$_9$, helps your brain get the blood it needs by inhibiting narrowing of the arteries in the neck. Studies also suggest that daily supplements of folic acid can reduce the likelihood of certain age-related brain problems, including dementia. Folic acid's main role is to maintain the cell's genetic code—its DNA, the master plan for cell reproduction. It also works with vitamin B$_{12}$ to form hemoglobin in red blood cells.

If your body isn't getting enough folic acid, you may suffer from forgetfulness. You'll also be at greater risk for dementia as you get older. You may also suffer from anemia, impaired growth, and abnormal digestive function. Be careful, though! Taking too much folic acid through supplements can mask a vitamin B$_{12}$ deficiency and could interfere with other medications. In the synthetic form—the form used to fortify foods and in supplements—folic acid has a UL (upper limit) of 1,000 micrograms (mcg) per day for adults over eighteen.

CELEBRATE YOUR STREAKS

Your brain, like your boss, prefers success to failure. When it has a success, it releases dopamine, a feel-good neurotransmitter. This actually helps you remember what you did right so you can repeat it. In contrast, when you fail, you don't get the nice dopamine reward—and so your brain can't quite figure out what you did wrong. Despite what all those motivation gurus say, failure doesn't actually teach you much. Success is how you learn. Researchers at MIT found that monkeys (which have brains a lot like ours) repeat the same mistakes over and over. Failure didn't change the monkey's behavior or help it do well on the next test. Success did.

Having a "streak"—where you successfully complete a certain habit or task repeatedly over a period of time—also causes your brain to release dopamine. The more successful you are over time, the more your brain wants you to be successful. So keep track of your brain-healthy habits. For example, every time you get some aerobic exercise, mark it on a calendar. When you review the calendar you'll see a series of successes and your brain will be motivated to continue succeeding. In other words, you can use your brain to help your brain stay healthy.

POWER UP WITH VITAMIN C

Vitamin C, an antioxidant, boosts the effectiveness of other antioxidants. It also helps your brain manufacture neurotransmitters such as dopamine and acetylcholine. In short, a daily dose of vitamin C can boost and maintain mental acuity. So important is vitamin C to proper brain function that it is being evaluated as a possible nutritional preventative for Alzheimer's disease.

From the point of view of your brain, vitamin C can help:

- Prevent mood swings
- Increase your intelligence
- Protect your brain against deterioration
- Guard against free radicals

Vitamin C prevents the oxidation of LDL or "bad" cholesterol and thereby decreases the risk for plaque formation, which can clog arteries and lead to a heart attack or stroke. Vitamin C protects vitamin E from oxidation and may also prevent blood vessels from constricting and thus cutting off blood supply to the brain. Studies have shown that 1,000 to 2,000 milligrams of vitamin C per day can help keep arteries healthy. Supplementing with 500 milligrams of vitamin C per day may lower blood pressure. So, load up on C!

Most fruits and vegetables provide vitamin C. Foods particularly high in C include hot chili peppers (raw), cantaloupe, sweet peppers, dark green leafy vegetables, tomatoes, kiwi, oranges, and mango.

Because vitamin C is a water-soluble vitamin, your body excretes the excess that may be consumed. Very large doses, though, could cause kidney stones, nausea, and diarrhea. The effects of taking large amounts over extended periods of time are not yet known. Vitamin C has a UL (upper limit) set at 2,000 milligrams per day for adults over eighteen.

BE A SOCIAL BUTTERFLY

Spending time with friends and loved ones makes you feel good. It increases your sense of happiness and well-being and decreases the likelihood of depression. Connecting with others can also help you ward off dementia. Research has shown the more isolated you are (socially speaking), the more likely you are to develop dementia. Other studies show that people who spend time socializing do better on memory tests and other learning. Keeping your brain strong and vital isn't just a one-person job—it takes a village. Throw a party, chat with your friends, share a meal with your kids. It'll help keep your brain youthful!

Here are some other ideas for socializing that don't require a lot of preparation and planning:

- Go to a religious service
- Take a class
- Talk with your neighbors
- Join a community group

Skype if you must but don't replace all of your in-person interactions with screen interactions. Being in the physical presence of other people provides the best boost for your brain.

OPT FOR OOLONG

Drinking oolong tea can help protect your brain. An oolong tea is not quite a green tea and not quite a black tea. It falls in between (being partly fermented). Oolong tea contains catechins, a type of flavonoid, which are known antioxidants (that is, they can help prevent free radicals from running rampant in your brain and hurting it). You can also find catechins in green teas. But many people prefer the taste of oolong tea, and they find that drinking too much green tea irritates the stomach.

One study showed that drinking catechins suppressed brain dysfunction—although mice, not humans, were the subjects of that study. Another study showed that catechins may work as chelators (substances that bond to a metal, in this case iron), and prevent excess metal from hurting the brain. Catechins are also known to protect the heart and blood vessels, potentially reducing the possibility of stroke.

According to one study, oolong tea contains polyphenols that help reduce stress. Another study showed that drinking oolong tea may help protect your brain from Alzheimer's—oolong tea may prevent certain toxins, such as a plaque protein, from killing brain cells. (You may recall that plaques are characteristic of brains with Alzheimer's.)

Oolong tea benefits your brain in another way—it generally contains more caffeine than green tea and can boost your alertness and your thinking skills. On the downside, too much caffeine can cause insomnia and make heart problems worse, so drink in moderation.

TAKE A DIP

Swimming is both fun and good for your brain. It's aerobic, which means it increases blood flow to your brain, improving cognitive function. But unlike other aerobic exercise that is done on land, swimming is done in the water (okay, maybe that was obvious). The increase resistance of water boosts the benefits. One study showed that swimming increased blood flow to cerebral arteries by about 10 to 15 percent as compared to aerobic exercise done on land. One study also showed that swimming may have antidepressive effects. Aerobic exercise in general can help generate new brain cells and repair damaged ones, and swimming fires up the whole brain: you use both hemispheres and all four lobes to swim. Keeping the entire brain active is one way to help improve cognition. Dive on in for brain benefits!

YOGA FOR LIFE

Yoga, an ancient Indian method of exercise, involves specific postures and breathing exercises. It increases strength, flexibility, circulation, posture, and overall body condition. And it also builds your brain. Its original purpose was to help practitioners gain control over the body and bring it into a state of balance in order to free the mind for spiritual contemplation—in other words, it was used as an aid to meditation. But yoga itself, separate from any meditation practice, can provide benefits to your brain.

A study performed at the University of Illinois found that just a single twenty-minute session of yoga can improve focus and the ability to retain new information. Other research shows that yoga can boost mood, reduce anxiety and inflammation, and lower stress levels. Separate MRI research shows that yoga practitioners who exercise regularly actually enlarge their brains as compared to people who don't practice yoga. One study showed enlargement in the areas of the brain associated with visualization, reducing stress, and directing attention.

If you're just starting out with yoga, it can be helpful to take a beginner class with a certified instructor who can show you the proper way to hold your poses and teach you the right breathing techniques.

CUT YOUR COMMUTE

A 2017 study by the University of Leicester is bad news for many drivers: spending more than two hours a day driving hurts your brain. One reason driving is bad for you is because it's a sedentary activity, and being sedentary is hard on your overall health (particularly your cardiovascular system). But it turns out that driving also shuts down your brain. Subjects in the study actually lost IQ points when they regularly drove long distances (such as daily commutes). People who did little or no driving had less decline in their cognitive powers. Researchers theorize that in addition to the sedentary problems associated with lots of driving, driving causes stress and fatigue, and the link between stress, fatigue, and cognitive decline is fairly well established. If your daily commute requires two or more hours a day behind the wheel, it's time to move closer to your work—or find a new job.

NIBBLE ON SOME CHOCOLATE

If you love chocolate, you already know eating it makes you happy. But did you know it's also good for your brain? A recent study found that people who ate chocolate at least once a week tended to have improved cognitive function. Those who ate more chocolate scored better on tests of memory and abstract thinking.

Cocoa beans contain an antioxidant called cocoa flavanols that may actually reverse some cognitive decline and help the brain work under demanding circumstances. But if you're going to eat chocolate for the brain benefits, don't skimp on quality. Since it's the cocoa beans that provide the protection for your brain, you want a chocolate that's higher in cocoa butter. Inexpensive chocolates are often blended with wax and contain very little real cocoa butter. Inexpensive brands are also made with partially hydrogenated palm oil, preservatives, and high amounts of sugar, which are bad for your overall nutrition. Quality chocolate, on the other hand, is made using real cocoa butter, the finest organic cocoa beans, and minimal sugar, making it an overall healthier choice. To counteract the sugar, saturated fats, and artificial flavorings in commercial candy bars, many people have turned to buying chocolate in its raw, organic form and making their own sweets.

GO WITH YOUR GUT

You may think your brain controls your body, but it doesn't do the job all by itself. Researchers are learning about the importance of the enteric nervous system—that is, the nerves that line your alimentary canal (mouth to butt). Your gut health doesn't just keep your body working smoothly, it affects your mood! And this goes beyond feeling bad about your upset tummy. You know how meeting someone special can give you "butterflies in your stomach"? That's an emotional signal from your enteric nervous system. In fact, the vast majority of the serotonin in your body is found in your belly. New understanding about how the gut affects mental and physical health has created the field of neurogastroenterology. What does that mean for you? Right now, researchers are still trying to figure out how the gut and the brain work together, but it's clear that taking care of gut issues, like treating irritable bowel syndrome, will help protect your brain and your mood.

STAY HYDRATED!

Simple dehydration—not drinking enough water—can cause the brain to react in strange ways. Symptoms of dehydration include fogginess, dizziness, and lack of concentration. Water is one of the most abundant substances in your body, and it is the nutrient your body needs in the greatest amounts—between 55 and 75 percent of your body weight is water. Water plays a vital role in almost every major function in the body. It transports nutrients and oxygen to the brain and carries waste products away from the body cells. The brain is 73 percent water, so if it's going to keep on functioning properly, that water has to be replenished.

The body has no provision to store water. On average, we lose about 10 cups of water each day just through perspiration, breathing, urination, and bowel movements. This does not include hot days or exercise sessions, when perspiration drains away even more water. The average adult needs to drink 8 to 12 cups of water each day. By the time you feel thirsty, you can already be on your way to becoming dehydrated. To be sure you are properly hydrated, check your urine to make sure it is clear or pale yellow (meaning diluted) rather than a darker yellow.

BELLY BREATHE

Most people breathe using their chests—taking shallow breaths using the intercostal muscles (between your ribs) to expand the chest. But abdominal, or diaphragmatic, breathing, also known as "belly" breathing, helps get more oxygen to your body—and your brain. With belly breathing, when air is taken in, the diaphragm contracts and the abdomen expands; when the air is exhaled, the reverse occurs. You can test yourself for abdominal breathing by laying your hand on your belly as you breathe. If it rises as you inhale, you are breathing with the diaphragm. If it lowers, you are breathing with the chest. To practice abdominal breathing, imagine that your in-breath is filling a balloon in your belly. When the balloon is full, exhale until you feel it is completely empty. Just a few of these deep abdominal breaths will bring relief from tension and ease stress. Research also suggests that the mere practice of focusing on your breathing helps calm the mind and sharpen attention. Deep breathing can also help elevate the production of neurotransmitters such as serotonin, making you feel happier.

LEAVE YOUR DESK FOR LUNCH

A recent survey showed that about half of workers eat lunch at their desk and many don't bother eating lunch at all. Are you one of those who dine by the glow of your computer screen? You should know that eating lunch at your desk is bad for your brain. In particular:

1. Being sedentary hurts your brain. Sitting too long in one place strains your cardiovascular system, may cause you to gain weight, and otherwise increases the likelihood that you'll end up with a stroke or other health problems.

2. Socializing with your coworkers is good for your brain. Instead of eating lunch alone, go out with your fellow wage-slaves—even the one you don't like very well. Not only does socializing make your brain happy, it will probably help you do better at work.

3. Taking a break feeds your brain. Give yourself something to look at besides your cubicle walls and something to think about other than that report you're working on. Coming back to your work refreshed and energized makes you more productive than slogging through it. Changing up your surroundings can help boost creativity and can help prevent stress and burnout.

PORTION IT OUT

You know that a healthy diet can help prevent all kinds of brain-related problems—everything from depression to dementia. Plus, a healthy diet will help you live longer. An important key to a healthy diet is not just watching what you eat but watching how much you eat. Studies have shown that overeating may reduce brain function, even causing memory loss. You don't need to weigh and measure all of your food each day, though. Once you understand what a serving size is and can visualize it, you'll be able to eyeball your dinner and rightsize your portions.

Keep in mind that portion sizes listed on package labels and in recipes don't necessarily reflect how you really eat, so in the beginning you may need to whip out the food scale to help calibrate your servings. Here are some shortcuts that will help you stay on track:

- A 3-ounce portion of cooked meat, poultry, or fish is about the size of a deck of playing cards.
- If you're eating rice or pasta, a good portion is about the size of a tennis ball.
- A ½ cup is about the size of three regular ice cubes.
- Also, remember this rule: 1 thumb tip equals 1 teaspoon, 3 thumb tips equal 1 tablespoon, and a whole thumb equals 1 ounce.

SKIP THE PESTICIDES

One reason organic foods are so popular is because shoppers know they are grown without many common fertilizers and pesticides. Research has established an association between the presence of heavy pesticides in food and problems in the brain development of fetuses and infants. And other studies show an association between pesticides and neurological changes in adults. So avoiding food that has been slathered in pesticides is (forgive us) a no-brainer. In addition to opting for organic food when possible, here are some other ways to reduce your consumption of those brain-unfriendly chemicals:

- Wash fruits and vegetables under running water—yes, even organic food, and even food you plan to peel.
- Dry the produce. This additional step helps eliminate some additional pesticides.
- Eat a variety of types of food to reduce your exposure to any one pesticide.
- Throw away the outer layer of leafy greens like lettuce and the skin of vegetables like onions.
- Trim fat from all meat because pesticides concentrate in fatty areas.
- Peel nonorganic fruits and vegetables that may have a high load of pesticide, such as potatoes and pears.

WASH YOUR HANDS

A number of studies have shown a connection between certain types of infections and stroke—that is, stroke can be a complication of another disease, such as flu or pneumonia. Preventing such infections in people who have risk factors for stroke is one obvious way to prevent stroke. A recent study by researchers at Columbia University showed that people with a medical history of more infections have more memory and other cognition problems than people with fewer infections. In other words, the more infections you have in your lifetime, the worse you do on tests of cognition. Chronic infections, such as those associated with herpes, were more problematic than acute infections, such as those associated with the common cold. Other studies have shown a link between infection and the progression of Alzheimer's. Although the reason why infections are connected to cognitive decline isn't clear, avoiding infection, particularly chronic infections, is one way to protect your brain health. So:

- Wash your hands, especially after toileting and before handling food.
- Keep your vaccinations up to date—adults often forget to stay current.
- Use condoms during sex (and practice other methods of safe sex).
- Don't share your toothbrush (or other personal care items).

BEAT ANXIETY

Almost everyone has experienced anxiety at least once, whether it was because of an upcoming test or an impending financial stressor. So you know that having anxiety can put a damper on how you enjoy life. Those who suffer from more chronic or unexplained sources of anxiety (generalized anxiety rather than situational anxiety) are at significant risk for depression, insomnia, and other brain-zapping conditions. Optimizing or boosting your anxiolytic (antianxiety) response can help. For example, taking supplements of gamma-aminobutyric acid (GABA), an amino acid that has a calming effect on the nervous system, can result in:

- Relief from anxiety, shakiness, or other nervous tension
- Improved sleep and recovery sensation
- Less mental chatter

According to the National Institutes of Health (part of the US Department of Health and Human Services), the following herbs have shown effectiveness in reducing anxiety:

- Ginkgo biloba
- Kava kava
- Valerian
- Theanine (found in green tea)
- Hops
- Lemon balm
- Skullcap
- Passionflower
- Chamomile

Most can be taken as a supplement or infused in a tea. If you have serious struggles with anxiety, discuss options with your doctor.

PUMP UP THE POSITIVITY

According to Daniel G. Amen, MD, author of the classic book *Making a Good Brain Great*, every thought releases brain chemicals. Positive, happy, hopeful, optimistic, and joyful thoughts produce yummy chemicals that create a sense of well-being and help your brain function at peak capacity; unhappy, miserable, negative, and dark thoughts have the opposite effect, effectively slowing down your brain and even creating depression. If you tend to focus on what can go wrong, or what is wrong, or how unhappy you are, or how someone hurt you, these negative thoughts can dim your brain's capacity to function. They sap the brain of its positive forcefulness. Dr. Amen suggests writing out negative thoughts to dispel their power over your brain.

GO GINKGO

The leaves of the ginkgo tree contain chemicals that can be used to treat memory and cognitive problems. In a study published in the *Journal of the American Medical Association*, researchers confirmed that people who take ginkgo extract for mild to severe dementia may see improvement in their abilities to remember and to interact socially. You can buy ginkgo biloba in both extract and capsule form. Buy a quality product and read the label. Look for products marked "24/6," an indication that the product contains 24 percent flavone glycosides and 6 percent terpenes, the chemicals that do the good work. Plan to take it for at least eight weeks before expecting improvement to show.

Ginkgo may interfere with antidepressant MAO-inhibitor drugs (monoamine oxidase inhibitors) such as phenelzine sulfate (Nardil) and tranylcypromine (Parnate). If you're on heart medication and want to take ginkgo, consult your doctor first. And be sure to stick to the recommended dose.

HUG IT OUT

A recent study by Carnegie Mellon University showed that feeling close to others, particularly through the sense of touch (such as from a hug), helps protect against stress-related diseases. People who had a high sense of connection had more hugs and less conflict, and when faced with exposure to an infection they developed less severe symptoms. People who felt less socially connected suffered more physically. Researchers in Sweden found that even in high-stress occupations, stress-related illnesses could be reduced by social connectedness. And researchers at UCLA have shown that the stress-reducing effects of such connectedness occur whether you give the love or get it.

In addition to protecting against illness, hugs boost your happiness. Physical contact with someone you care about reduces anxiety levels, lowers cortisol (the stress hormone), and encourages the brain to produce oxytocin and dopamine, feel-good neurotransmitters that help lift your mood. Researchers have even concluded that the optimum hug is at least twenty seconds long. Researchers have also found that hugging your pet has similar effects, so even if you live alone, you can get your daily dose of hugging from Fido.

WATCH OUT FOR THE WHITE STUFF

Glucose, a form of sugar, powers every action in your body. Your brain needs it to function—in fact, it uses up half of the sugar energy your body produces. Without enough sugar, your brain gets lethargic and slows down. But scientists are finding out that too much sugar in your diet also causes brain trouble in the form of reduced cognitive function. Eat too many candy bars and you won't think as well. Too much sugar makes you forgetful and less able to learn things. It can also make you prone to anxiety and depression. The key is to eat sugar in moderation. The typical American diet is packed with sugar, much of it hidden (it's in everything from ketchup to salad dressing to pasta sauce). Nutrition experts agree that Americans need to cut back on sugar consumption.

Sugars are simple carbohydrates that the body uses as a source of energy. During digestion, all carbohydrates break down into sugar, or blood glucose. Some sugars occur naturally, such as in dairy products (as lactose) and fruits (as fructose). Other sugars are added for taste. Most foods containing added sugars provide calories but little in the way of essential nutrients, such as fiber, vitamins, and minerals. It's better to eat fruit, which in addition to fructose has healthy substances such as vitamin C, vitamin A, potassium, folic acid, antioxidants, phytochemicals, and fiber, just to name a few. Most fruits have no fat, and all are cholesterol free.

There is no current recommended dietary allowance (RDA) for sugar, but experts recommend that about 55 to 60 percent of total calories in your diet should come from carbohydrates, with less than 10 percent coming from simple sugars like lactose and fructose. The American Heart Association recommends no more than 6 teaspoons of sugar per day for women and 9 teaspoons for men.

GO NUTS

The folks at Harvard did a study that showed that eating nuts can lead to increased life span. That's at least in part because nuts are good for your brain. Nuts are high in fat but they contain minerals, fiber, and nice amounts of protein, along with omega-3 fatty acids. Studies show they can improve cognitive performance and slow decline. Nuts are high in calories, and so they should be eaten in moderation; think of a serving as a tablespoon or two. Look for nuts that are unsalted; it's not important whether they are roasted or raw, although dry roasting is preferable to oil roasting. Nuts are great sprinkled on foods high in vitamin C, such as fruit and vegetables, because the vitamin C increases the body's absorption of the iron in nuts.

The four best nuts for brain health:

- Walnuts
- Almonds
- Hazelnuts
- Peanuts

STEP UP YOUR SEROTONIN

Serotonin is a neurotransmitter that helps your brain communicate with your body. Low serotonin levels are associated with mood problems like anxiety and depression. On the other hand, too much serotonin causes nausea and diarrhea.

Your body creates serotonin from the tryptophan you get from food. (The first step is for the body to convert tryptophan to 5-HTP [5-hydroxy-tryptophan], which is then converted to serotonin.) Thus, the more tryptophan you eat, the more serotonin your brain will create. Serotonin itself won't cross the blood-brain barrier, so taking serotonin itself, such as in a supplement, doesn't help.

Foods that provide tryptophan (and thereby stimulate production of 5-HTP) include white-meat turkey, ground beef, cottage cheese, chicken thighs, pumpkin seeds, milk, and almonds. You may remember from Thanksgiving that too much tryptophan from the turkey will make you tired, so as with everything, moderation is key. You can also stimulate production of serotonin in your brain by breathing deeply and by getting a massage.

LOWER THE PRESSURE

If you have hypertension or are at risk for it, reducing your blood pressure will help your brain. High blood pressure increases the risk of cognitive decline, because high blood pressure reduces blood flow to the brain. This causes changes in your brain, which can be anything from mild confusion to severe memory loss. High blood pressure can also create the conditions, such as blood clots and weakening of the arteries, that cause stroke. Protect your brain by keeping your blood pressure numbers in check. Here are some steps to take:

- First, find out if you have hypertension or are at risk. Many people don't realize they have high blood pressure.
- Eat right and exercise.
- Reduce stress.
- Eliminate sodium.
- Keep tabs on your blood pressure at home.
- Use prescription medications to lower blood pressure if needed.

USE THE PLACEBO EFFECT

According to Daniel G. Amen, MD, author of *Making a Good Brain Great*, placebos (inert substances with no physiological effects or medicinal properties) are astonishingly effective. He noted that 150 years ago, doctors relied more on their relationship with their patients and the administration of placebos to treat illnesses. Many patients improved, based on how much they trusted their doctors and how much they believed that they would get well.

Recent studies have shown that the placebo effect works for diseases such as depression, anxiety, and Parkinson's (although not for cancer or Alzheimer's). One researcher theorizes that expectations influence how well placebos work. For example, Parkinson's results from the lack of dopamine in the brain. And our brains produce dopamine in response to expectations. The takeaway? Your mind may be able to help you think yourself well!

MUNCH ON PUMPKIN SEEDS

Pumpkin seeds, also known as pepitas, nestle in the core of the pumpkin encased in a white-yellow husk. These super seeds contain a number of minerals, such as zinc, magnesium, manganese, iron, copper, and phosphorus, along with proteins, monounsaturated fat, and the omega-3 and omega-6 fatty acids—all of which aid the brain in different ways. They also contain the amino acid glutamate, which helps the brain produce the antianxiety chemical GABA (gamma-aminobutyric acid). Pumpkin seeds help improve memory and focus. You can use pumpkin seeds as a garnish, add them to granola, or roast them and eat them by the handful. If you're not a huge fan of the seeds, pumpkin seed oil has many similar benefits.

TAP INTO YOUR CREATIVITY

You probably think the best time to tap into your creativity—to solve a problem or produce a work of art—is when you're sharpest and most alert. But research says that's not true. In fact, people are generally more creative when they're tired (not exhausted, just tired). When you're tired, your brain is not as vigilant about filtering out background information—thoughts and stimulus that it normally wouldn't attend to. But creative work requires connecting different ideas together or thinking in new ways, which is more likely to happen when you're tired. Creativity also requires imagination, which the thinking frontal lobe tends to suppress—except when it's tired. Looking for new insights? Tackle them just before bedtime.

CUT THE FAT

Your brain is about 60 percent fat and uses 20 percent of your body's metabolic energy, so it's not too surprising that you need some fat in your diet. Without it, your nervous system and metabolism aren't able to function normally. Fat helps carry, absorb, and store the fat-soluble vitamins (A, D, E, and K) in your bloodstream. But a diet that's too high in fat can damage synapses in the hippocampus area of the brain, the part that affects memory and learning. Moderate your fat intake by using some of the following tips:

- Choose low-fat or fat-free dairy products.
- Use low-fat dressings and limit buttermilk, ranch, and blue cheese dressings.
- Use nonstick cooking sprays or nonstick pans and avoid frying anything in oil.
- Trim excess fat and skin from all meat and poultry.
- Choose foods based on amount of total fat and type of fat.
- Watch for hidden fats: pizza toppings, fried foods, ice cream, high-fat meat (salami, bologna, bratwurst, hot dogs, pepperoni, sausage, bacon, and spare ribs), cakes, cookies, macaroni salad, potato salad, and coleslaw.
- Limit your intake of red meat; opt for poultry, fish, or nonmeat dishes more often.
- Limit your use of cream sauces on pastas; use marinara or other tomato-based toppings instead.

STOP SNORING

Snoring may be a sign of obstructive sleep apnea, which means you're having trouble breathing as you sleep. Apnea is bad for your brain, as it causes sleep deprivation, which leads to memory loss. Sleep apnea can also change the structure of your brain, damage neurons, and impact your ability to think clearly and make decisions. The good news is that much of the damage is reversible as long as the apnea is treated. If you suspect you have sleep apnea, request an evaluation from your healthcare provider and get treatment.

SNACK SMART

Most dietitians agree that eating multiple small meals throughout the day is much healthier than eating only the usual three large meals. Small meals keep the flow of nutrients to your body going, and the brain especially needs these nutrients to function well. Research has shown that a steady supply of glucose is healthier for the brain than having it come in spurts.

Choosing snacks wisely can help fuel your body (especially your brain) between meals, give you an energy boost, and add to your total intake of essential nutrients for the day. Snacking can also help to take the edge off hunger between meals. The longer you wait between meals, the more you tend to eat at the next meal. Here are some tips for smart snacking:

- Choose snacks that are lower in fat and nutrient rich.
- Make snacks part of your eating plan for the day instead of thinking of them as extras.
- Make snacking a conscious activity, not a mindless face-stuffing situation.
- Eat snacks in smaller portions, not meal-size ones.

Try some of these smart snacks as part of your healthy eating plan:

- ½ bagel with peanut butter
- Raw vegetables with low-fat or fat-free dressing
- Fruit yogurt topped with low-fat granola cereal
- Low-fat cottage cheese topped with fresh fruit
- A piece of fresh fruit
- Light microwave popcorn
- Pita bread stuffed with fresh veggies and low-fat dressing
- Low-fat string cheese
- Whole-grain cereal and fat-free milk
- Vegetable juice

IT'S ALL IN THE ATTITUDE

Doing challenging work—like figuring out a calculus problem—seems to take a lot of energy, and so it makes your brain feel tired. Spending the same time on *Facebook* looking at cat pictures doesn't seem as mentally demanding, because your brain doesn't use nearly the same amount of energy to do that. Right? Not so fast.

Stress contributes to the feeling of exhaustion you might have after doing challenging work, such as taking a calculus test, where you are worried about your grade and are anxious about your performance. So it's true that under certain circumstances doing challenging work tires your brain more than easy tasks. But research shows that it's basically your attitude that makes the difference. In other words, you just think that solving the calculus problem is more tiring than looking at cat pictures. As far as how much energy your brain actually uses? There's not a lot of difference between the two activities.

One study showed that the expectation of mental fatigue actually predicted it. That is, if a person thinks a task will be hard, it often is. So imagine if you changed your attitude. Instead of letting your brain trick you into thinking it's exhausted, remind yourself that those cat pictures are just as hard on it.

FIND THE RIGHT FAT

You know that your brain needs fat—in moderation!—to function. Ideally, you should eat healthy fats. But the truth is most American diets are overloaded with unhealthy fats. These are the saturated, hydrogenated, and partially hydrogenated (trans) fats found in all commercial baked goods, margarines, and processed foods. Saturated fats are usually solid at room temperature and can be found in well-marbled meat, butter, whole-milk cheese, ice cream, egg yolks, and fatty cuts of beef, pork, and lamb. Certain vegetable oils, such as palm, palm kernel, and coconut oils, are also saturated. According to the Alzheimer's Research and Prevention Foundation, the ideal prevention diet includes:

- 20 percent "good" fats, such as extra-virgin olive oil
- 40 percent lean protein, such as fish, chicken, turkey, and soy
- 40 percent complex carbohydrates, like fresh fruits and vegetables, whole grains, and legumes
- Lots of superfoods, including blueberries, spinach, and seaweed

What are the "good" fats? Here are some to try:

- Avocado oil
- Flaxseed oil
- Olive oil
- Sesame oil
- Walnut oil

KICK OUT CHOLESTEROL

Your body needs cholesterol to protect nerve cells and make it easier for them to send out the electric discharges that keep you functioning. About 25 percent of the body's cholesterol is found in the brain. However, you don't need to consume it: your body can produce all the cholesterol it needs to function.

Dietary cholesterol comes directly from animal foods, such as egg yolks, meat, poultry, fish, seafood, and whole-milk dairy products. Consuming these foods can raise your cholesterol levels higher than is healthy. Saturated fat raises your LDL (bad) cholesterol level more than anything else in your diet. Trans fats also raise blood cholesterol. Foods high in saturated fat generally contain substantial amounts of dietary cholesterol. Here are a few ways you can lower the cholesterol in your diet:

- Buy lower-fat versions of foods, such as dressings, mayonnaise, margarine, and cream cheese.

- Eat no more than four egg yolks per week. One large egg has about 186 milligrams of cholesterol, but it's all in the yolk—the egg white has no cholesterol. Try substituting two egg whites for one whole egg in baked goods or using an egg substitute.

- Limit organ meat, such as liver. They are nutritious but also very high in cholesterol.

- Enjoy seafood—prepared in a low-fat way—as your main meal a few times per week.

- Make vegetarian meals occasionally. Meals with beans or soy products as the main protein source have cholesterol-lowering qualities.

HERB YOURSELF UP

Herbal remedies have become immensely popular as a natural alternative to pharmaceutical drugs. Using herbal remedies can promote memory function and general neurological function. Herbs are also sometimes used to treat depression, lethargy, attention deficit, and other issues. Always consult with your physician before ingesting herbal remedies, particularly if you are pregnant.

When buying packaged herbal products, choose a reliable brand and follow the manufacturer's directions concerning dosage. Buy only from reputable manufacturers. The label should include the company's address, batch and lot numbers, expiration date, and recommended dosage.

Consider using the following herbs to help support brain function:

- Energy—fo-ti, ginseng, and gotu kola
- Fatigue—capsicum (cayenne), ginseng, American ginseng and red deer antler (combination), gotu kola, and oats
- Insomnia—catnip, chamomile, hops, lady's slipper, skullcap, and valerian
- Memory—astragalus, calamus, cayenne, dong quai, ginger, ginkgo biloba leaf extract, ginseng, gotu kola, and red deer antler
- Mental health—cayenne, ginseng, and gotu kola
- Nervousness—betony, catnip, chamomile, European vervain, hops, lady's slipper, mistletoe, passionflower, pulsatilla, red sage (for nervous headache), skullcap, and valerian
- Stress—alfalfa, chamomile, ginseng, gotu kola, hops, kelp, lady's slipper, passionflower, and valerian

TAKE A TRIP DOWN MEMORY LANE

One way to stimulate your memory and give it a workout is to take a trip down memory lane. Remember a past experience by looking at old photos, watching a video, or talking with a friend. Go through your *Facebook* timeline. Nostalgia actually feels good for your brain, even if you're young and the events are fairly recent. That feel-good trigger makes you feel more optimistic and positive about the future. One recent study showed that digging into your long-term memory also helps improve overall brain function and even stimulates your short-term memory. In other words, a little visit to the past can help your brain deal with the present.

FACE DOWN YOUR PHOBIAS

A phobia is an unreasonable, compulsive, persistent fear of any specific type of situation (such as flying) or thing (such as spiders). Having to face something that you fear can produce a phobic anxiety attack. Such an attack may include a number of physical reactions, such as heart palpitations, breathlessness, weakness, an uncontrollable feeling of terror, and hysterical screaming. Anxiety and phobias are closely related. Stress and unresolved conflicts can lead to a chronic state of anxiety. Individuals suffering from chronic anxiety may develop a phobia as a safety net. As long as these individuals avoid the phobia-producing situation or thing, they can repress their ever-present anxiety and lead a fairly stable life. However, when the person encounters the fear-inducing object, the repressed anxiety may erupt into a phobic anxiety attack. If you have a phobia, therapy and meditation can help you face and conquer your phobias and lead you to greater peace of mind and a calmer brain.

TRY SOME SAGE ADVICE

For centuries, it was believed that sage could be used to enhance memory. Now studies have shown that this belief is, in fact, true. Eating sage seems to help produce acetylcholine, which is a chemical in the brain that aids memory. Studies have shown that small amounts of sage help with recall and concentration. It's also an antioxidant that will help your brain get rid of those pesky free radicals. Some researchers are looking at sage in relationship to treating more serious brain disorders such as Alzheimer's.

In addition to this, of course, it's delicious in foods like omelets, spaghetti sauce, turkey (or really, any kind of poultry), and a lot more. Sprinkle it on with a generous hand and your brain will reap the benefits.

REDUCE YOUR BLOOD SUGAR

Your brain doesn't exist on its own—it's part of your body. And unlike in Vegas, what happens in other parts of your body doesn't necessarily stay there. For example, people with type 2 diabetes are known to be at increased risk for dementia, including Alzheimer's, although research has not yet determined the specific mechanisms for why this is so. Even being prediabetic (insulin resistant) is a risk factor. Researchers haven't proven that controlling your blood sugar will reduce your likelihood of dementia, but it's a safe step to take given the strong correlation. At worst, by controlling your blood sugar you'll reduce your chance of having diabetes (or get it under better control), which is a legitimate goal all by itself. Controlling your blood sugar is a lot like protecting your brain—you must eat right, exercise, drink enough water, and control stress. So that you can effectively address your particular situation, you should work with your healthcare provider to monitor your blood sugar levels.

CHEW GUM

Your dentist may frown on it, but chewing gum can benefit your brain. If you've ever chomped on gum before an anxiety-producing situation, like taking a test, then you already know it can help relieve stress. But chewing gum can also improve cognitive function. Chewing it increases blood flow to your brain, enhancing your ability to think. It can also make you more alert, particularly if you're sleepy. One study showed that chewing gum quickened reaction times and made it easier for subjects to form new memories. And, fortunately, chewing gum does not have the downside of multitasking—it doesn't distract you from whatever task is at hand. However, the benefits of gum chewing require you to keep chewing. Once you stop, the benefits disappear. Keep your dentist happy and pick a gum that uses xylitol rather than sugar as the sweetener.

DITCH THE TRANS FATS

Manmade trans fats are hard on your brain. What are trans fats? They're artificially produced solid fats. The hydrogenation process (introduction of hydrogen) causes the atomic structure of a substance to change so that what was once a liquid can now remain a solid at room temperature. Why would anyone do that to a bottle of vegetable oil? Well, around World War II, scientists developed hydrogenated fats and oils to provide a longer shelf life for foods that were being transported around the world for soldiers. Butter goes rancid quickly, but margarine doesn't. The problem is that research has shown that trans fats can increase LDL (bad) cholesterol and lower HDL (good) cholesterol—the exact opposite of what most people need! Not only that, trans fats disrupt the production of energy in the mitochondria (the energy factories) of brain cells. Trans fats may be even more harmful than saturated fats and hydrogenated oils (which don't contain trans fats). In general, most health experts these days recommend avoiding trans fats altogether. If you must have a buttery spread, the good news is that there are margarines on the market today that are low in both saturated fats and trans fats. Many of these margarines are called "spreads" because they are less than 80 percent oil. (That is, the more solid a margarine is, the more saturated fat and trans fat it contains.) When looking for margarine spreads, look for one with no more than 30 percent fat from saturated fat plus trans fat. Less than 20 percent is even better. Look for words such as *trans-free*, which means the spread has no more than half a gram of trans fat per serving. But be sure the manufacturers are not replacing trans fats with saturated fats. In moderation, such spreads can be part of a brain-healthy lifestyle.

PUT SOME ALFALFA IN YOUR LIFE

You probably haven't considered adding alfalfa to your diet, but for a healthy brain you really should. This herb, which takes its name from the Arabic meaning "the father of all foods," contains a lot of the nutrients your brain needs to keep going.

Scientists have discovered that alfalfa can help in the treatment of heart disease, cancer, and stroke—three of the top five causes of death in the United States. Alfalfa leaves—which contain its real healing properties—are rich in minerals and other nutrients, including calcium, magnesium, potassium, and beta-carotene. Consuming alfalfa may reduce "bad" cholesterol. Alfalfa is commonly eaten in sprouts. Alfalfa leaf is on the FDA's list of herbs generally regarded as safe, but it should be used in medicinal amounts only with your doctor's approval. If you experience any side effects—such as upset stomach or diarrhea—stop use. If you have an autoimmune problem, avoid alfalfa seeds entirely.

STUDY, STUDY, STUDY

Research has shown that the more education you receive, the better your mental acuity—and the longer you will retain it. Take a class on a topic that challenges your thought processes rather than something with which you're already familiar. Most community colleges and universities offer continuing education classes on a wide variety of subjects, and many sessions are held at night to accommodate people who work during the day. Choose a challenging but interesting subject, something that forces you to think or that flexes brain cells you haven't used for eons.

If you are planning a trip to a museum, study the topic of the exhibit you are going to see ahead of time. For example, if you'll be visiting an art museum, brush up on art history and learn about the artists and the eras. See how much you can memorize, and then use your knowledge to enhance the experience. You can also do this process for stargazing, attending classical music concerts, opera, theater, and so on. Give it a try when going to a basketball game or skiing. You'll stimulate your brain (and maybe impress your friends).

KILL THE CLUTTER

Maybe you've heard that an untidy desk is the sign of a creative mind. Perhaps this is the very excuse you use for living with untidiness. But clutter is actually bad for your brain. It can make you feel anxious and overwhelmed. If clutter is all around you, your brain gets overstimulated as it tries to figure out if there is something meaningful in the mess. Because your brain is attending to the ninety-two things in the background, it can't focus on the task at hand. Clutter signals that there is work to do, making it difficult to relax. Clutter can also create stress when you misplace something and have to dig around to find it.

Keep in mind that we're not talking about hoarding here, which is a distinct mental health problem. We're just talking about the general untidiness that comes from having a busy life and no real recognition of how stressful clutter actually is. Here are some very simple steps you can take to clear the clutter—and your mind:

- Close doors. If you can't see it, your brain will stop worrying about it. Use cabinets, boxes, and drawers to hide the clutter.
- Get in the habit of putting things back where they belong.
- Enlist a friend to help you declutter. They'll be more ruthless about your stuff than you are.
- Don't try to do too much at once. Clearing clutter is a decision-making process, and the more you decide, the worse your judgment gets.

SUPPLEMENT YOUR AMINO ACIDS

Several studies on phosphatidylserine, an amino acid that your body uses in building cell membranes, show how important it is to our mental health. A study reported in *Clinical Interventions in Aging* found that supplementation with 300 milligrams a day of soybean-derived phosphatidylserine significantly improved memory recognition, memory recall, executive functions, and mental flexibility. Some of the most notable benefits of supplementation include, but are not limited to:

- Improved memory
- Increased concentration
- Increased attention
- Improved learning ability
- Boost in mood (primarily fights depression)
- Preventing damage from exercise and stress
- Balanced cortisol

DOODLE

Even if you have no artistic talent, doodling can be a creative outlet that stimulates your brain. The act of drawing forces your brain to become attentive, to truly perceive what you're trying to capture with your pencil. But what's less well-known is that doodling—long dismissed as a mindless activity that you do while you're doing something else—has brain benefits. A study published in *Applied Cognitive Psychology* showed that doodling helped people remember information, particularly if the information was tedious. In other words, the doodling helped people focus their minds. Without doodling, their minds were likely to wander and subjects did not pay attention to what they were learning. According to one researcher, doodling is a type of visual language that can help people access ideas and thoughts they wouldn't otherwise have, so it's a boon to creativity as well.

GET YOUR COMPLEX CARBS

Carbohydrates are your body's main source of energy, especially for the brain and nervous system. Your brain uses a lot of carbohydrates during the day. If you don't get enough complex carbs, you can start to feel light-headed and find it hard to concentrate. You'll find carbohydrates in almost every type of food except meat. Carbohydrates are either simple carbohydrates (sugars) or complex carbohydrates (starches). Sugars are carbohydrates in their simplest form, such as fructose found in fruit. Complex carbohydrates are basically many simple sugars linked together. Complex carbohydrates are found in foods such as grains, pasta, rice, vegetables, breads, legumes, nuts, and seeds.

Your body converts all carbohydrates into glucose to be used as energy for the body, including your brain. Glucose circulating in your bloodstream is known as blood sugar. This sugar enters your body's cells, where it is converted to energy. Since simple carbohydrates, or simple sugars, are already in their simplest form, they go straight into the bloodstream. Complex carbohydrates require digestive enzymes to convert them into glucose. Some glucose is used immediately for energy and some is stored in the liver and muscles in the form of glycogen. By eating complex carbs, you can help your body and brain function at high capacity without causing spikes in your blood sugar levels.

Healthy adults should consume approximately 50 percent of their total daily calories from carbohydrates. That means filling more than half of your plate with carbohydrate-rich foods such as grains, vegetables, and beans. The idea is to eat larger amounts of complex carbohydrates and smaller portions of protein and fat.

PACK IN THE (SWEET) POTATOES

In addition to providing lots of general health benefits, sweet potatoes are good for optimum brain health. Including sweet potatoes in the diet has been shown to improve memory and reduce the possibility of Alzheimer's down the road. For about 100 calories per ½-cup serving you get a huge amount of health-building nutrients. The bright orange flesh of the sweet potato contains carotenoids that help stabilize your blood sugar, aiding your metabolism. Sweet potatoes have four times the US recommended dietary allowance (RDA) for beta-carotene when eaten with the skin on. In fact, it would take 20 cups of broccoli to provide the 38,000 IUs (international units) of beta-carotene (which converts to vitamin A) that is available in 1 cup of cooked sweet potatoes. They are also a source of vitamin E, vitamin B_6, potassium, and iron, plus they're fat-free. Cup for cup, sweet potatoes have been found to provide as much fiber as oatmeal.

BECOME YOUR OWN GPS

A recent study showed that London black-cab drivers—who must navigate thousands of streets and bring tourists to thousands of landmarks—have structural differences in their brains related to spatial memory as compared to a control group of bus drivers. The bus drivers follow a set, preplanned route, whereas the cabbies rely on their brains and their memory (no GPS!) to get from place to place.

But you don't have to be a London cab driver to strengthen your spatial memory. You can stimulate it by driving or walking in a new city using maps rather than GPS. You'll also build up your problem-solving and decision-making skills. If you don't travel much, try taking a new route at home in order to achieve a similar benefit.

AVOID FORMALDEHYDE

Formaldehyde is used in the manufacture of a wide number of household products, including plywood, particle board, paneling, countertops, flooring, and carpeting. While it serves useful functions, overexposure to it can create big problems for your brain. A study in the *International Journal of Anatomy and Physiology* reported issues from formaldehyde poisoning range from headaches to brain cancer.

Household products that include formaldehyde often send it out as fumes, resulting in chronic respiratory problems. Millions of Americans are affected. If you live in a newly built tract home, condominium, townhouse, or mobile home, you risk greater exposure because these places tend to use more products known to contain formaldehyde. If you suffer from unexplained respiratory problems, headaches, or other mysterious symptoms, you could be the victim of formaldehyde exposure. To reduce your risk, air out items known to contain high levels of formaldehyde, such as new furniture and carpeting, before bringing them into your home.

CHOOSE WHOLE GRAINS

In addition to choosing complex carbs over simple sugars, you should make sure that at least some of these complex carbs are from whole grains. Your body digests whole grains more slowly than refined grains, which provides your body with a steady stream of glucose, something that helps keep your brain running smoothly.

Whole-grain foods supply vitamin E and B vitamins such as folic acid as well as minerals like magnesium, iron, and zinc. Whole grains (like whole wheat) are rich in fiber and higher in other important nutrients. In fact, eating plenty of whole-grain breads, bran cereals, and other whole-grain foods can easily provide half of your fiber needs for an entire day. Avoid refined grains, such as white bread and white rice. "Whole grain" describes the entire edible part of any grain, including wheat, corn, oats, and rice. Refined grains go through a milling process in which parts of the grain are removed. In refined grains, many of the essential nutrients are lost in processing. Some nutrients are added back in, or the product is enriched, but this usually does not include all of the nutrients that were lost. To make sure you eat more whole-grain foods rather than refined grains, look for words such as *whole grain, whole wheat, rye, bulgur, brown rice, oatmeal, whole oats, pearl barley,* and *whole-grain corn* as one of the first listed ingredients on a food label.

RELAX!

In the late 1960s, Harvard cardiologist Herbert Benson, MD, discovered that relaxation methods could counterbalance both the psychological and physiological changes caused by the body's fight-or-flight response. He called this the "relaxation response." Benson's tests showed that people who simply sat quietly for ten or fifteen minutes with their minds focused on a single word, idea, or thought could markedly change their physiology. These subjects decreased their metabolism, slowed their heart and respiratory rates, and exhibited brain waves of the alpha-theta pattern, which indicates deep relaxation (but not sleep). Benson showed that the relaxation response, no matter how it was achieved, caused bodily transformations. It caused heart rate, breathing rate, muscle tension, and oxygen consumption to fall below resting levels; it encouraged decreases in blood pressure; and it helped the waking brain shift into the slower patterns associated with reverie and daydreaming. These slightly altered states of consciousness promote healing in the same way sleep does. If you focus your mind and relax, you, too, can achieve these results.

GO NATURAL

Medical professionals specially trained in natural medicine, called naturopaths, are fully licensed MDs who generally recommend natural approaches to the treatment of health problems, rather than relying on invasive procedures or pharmaceutical options. They're especially helpful in approaching the body holistically, seeing the connections between brain health and the health of the rest of you. To find a naturopath in your area, visit the website of the American Association of Naturopathic Physicians (www.naturopathic.org). Naturopathic doctors' fees can range from $35 to $175 for an initial consultation, but you can expect naturopathic practitioners to spend considerably more time with you than other MDs, especially those who work for HMOs. And naturopathic doctors typically offer the same level of professionalism as do regular MDs.

USE THE EIGHT SECOND RULE

Face it. We all have so much information coming at us that it's a wonder we remember any of it! But this simple trick will help you move information from your short-term (working) memory into your long-term memory: think about the information for at least eight seconds. You can't assume that because something flashed across your mind, you'll remember it. If a piece of information doesn't go into your long-term storage banks, you won't remember it. Researchers have found that it takes at least eight seconds for something new to get stored in our long-term memories, where we can retrieve it. So, concentrate on new information, repeat it a few times, then quiz yourself.

EAT THE RAINBOW

Eating a variety of fruits and vegetables is key to a healthy diet and a healthy brain. Different types of fruits and vegetables are rich in different essential nutrients, such as vitamins, minerals, and fiber—not to mention micronutrients. Eating a variety of foods ensures a greater intake of these essential nutrients. Aim to try different types throughout the week. One tip: make sure the food on your plate includes lots of different colors. If everything's white or beige—potato, rice, chicken—that's a recipe for disaster. Another tip: each week, pick up a new fruit or vegetable at the grocery store or farmers' market and try it in a variety of dishes. Don't keep relying on the same five or six old favorites.

Whether you choose fresh, frozen, canned, dried, or juice, your brain will benefit. But remember that juices and canned fruits do not provide as much fiber as the other types, so it is best to eat the whole fruit or vegetable more often. Eat at least two servings of fruit and three servings of vegetables per day.

LEARN A LANGUAGE

Being multilingual has many benefits for your brain. Learning a foreign language is mentally challenging because it requires the thoughtful assimilation of new information and a strong memory. Your brain benefits when you struggle with those verbs, pore over grammatical structure, force yourself to practice speaking the target language at every opportunity, and stick with it even when it seems futile. The minute it feels like your brain is stretching, you're already succeeding. Once you've learned a new language, reward yourself with a vacation to a country where it is spoken. Not only can you practice speaking the new language, but you can learn more about the country's culture. Your brain will thank you.

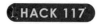

EMBRACE DISCOMFORT

One important way to stimulate your brain and get it working hard is to push yourself out of your comfort zone. This can mean learning new skills and information, meeting new people, and making great memories. You could:

- Travel somewhere you've never been
- Go to a meeting of an organization you don't know much about
- Say hello to people in your neighborhood
- Go on a dating site
- Try food you've never tasted before

Any one of these things—and lots of others—will stimulate your brain and keep it active and happy.

FOCUS ON THE PRESENT

Practitioners of yoga, transcendental meditation, and Buddhism all know that being mindful contributes to having a happier, less stressful life. Mindfulness is often practiced in association with meditation, where one is mindful of one's breathing and one's thoughts. More generally, the practice of mindfulness helps train the mind to avoid negative patterns and thought processes, vicious circles of failure, low self-esteem, and even the perception of chronic pain as an intensely negative experience. The brain is a complex and amazing organ, and mindfulness can teach you to harness your mind's power, integrate your mind and body, and feed your hungry spirit. The key is not to spend too much time regretting the past or worrying about the future. Instead, focus intently on what you are doing in the present moment.

ENJOY THE SOUND OF MUSIC

Scientific research suggests our brains are hardwired to appreciate music. In fact, some researchers say that listening to music can help people who suffer from neurodegenerative diseases like Parkinson's. Elena Mannes, author of *The Power of Music*, says that music stimulates more parts of the brain than anything else we do. This is why she believes music therapy is so important for anyone who has lost brain function.

Researchers have found that the same pleasure centers of the brain that are positively stimulated by food and sex are also affected by music. Any music that sends chills up your spine has a direct effect upon your mood. When you use music that is particularly stimulating to you in a positive way, you can experience a host of positive effects that include elevating your mood and feeling more content, relaxed, energized, or turned on.

Your choice of music is your own. But whether you like Beethoven or the Beatles, hip hop or country and western, sit back and listen to some music. Your brain will thank you.

EAT BETA

Beta-carotene, a fat-soluble antioxidant, is what makes carrots and sweet potatoes orange. Your body converts it to vitamin A. In addition to carrots and sweet potatoes, you'll find beta-carotene in liver, milk, butter, spinach, squash, broccoli, yams, tomatoes, cantaloupe, peaches, and grains. All of these foods are good for your brain because, as it turns out, beta-carotene reduces the risk of cognitive decline. One long-term study showed significant improvement in memory, recognition, and verbal skills in people who ate beta-carotene versus those who took a placebo (inert substance). Making sure you eat beta-rich foods boosts your overall health as well.

KICK UP YOUR MAGNESIUM

Magnesium, a mineral, is an absolute must for proper brain function. It aids neuron metabolism and boosts the effectiveness of certain antioxidants. Magnesium may also play a role in the prevention of Alzheimer's disease. Studies show that the brains of most Alzheimer's patients are deficient in magnesium but excessively high in calcium. In healthy brains, the two minerals have a relatively equal ratio. Higher magnesium intakes have been linked to a lower risk of stroke.

Magnesium can be found in a wide variety of foods. The best sources include legumes, almonds, avocados, toasted wheat germ, wheat bran, fish, seafood, fruits, fruit juice, pumpkin seeds, and whole grains. Green vegetables, especially cooked spinach, can be good sources too.

Magnesium deficiency can result from an increase in urine output (like that caused by diuretics), poorly controlled diabetes, and alcoholism. People who suffer from migraine headaches may also be magnesium deficient. In one study, migraine patients who took 600 milligrams of magnesium per day for twelve weeks went from three attacks per month down to two. Migraine patients who were given the placebo noticed no change in the number of headaches.

Too much magnesium is not harmful unless the mineral is not excreted properly due to disorders such as kidney disease. The UL (upper limit) for magnesium is 350 milligrams per day for adults over eighteen.

PLAY VIDEO GAMES

It doesn't matter if it's on a Wii, Xbox, Switch, or PlayStation, playing video games can improve your brain as well as build hand-eye coordination and spatial visualization (the ability to imagine moving and rotating two- and three-dimensional objects). Researchers in Belgium analyzed the brains of 150 teenagers. They found that the ones who played video games regularly had more cells in the left ventral striatum of their brains—the part of the brain connected to emotions and behavior. Other studies have shown that those who play action video games build stronger perception, attention, and cognition skills than non–game players. So plug in a Call of Duty game and get going!

GET FABULOUS PHOSPHORUS

Phosphorus is an important component of human bones. In fact, it is the second most abundant mineral in the body and the second most important element after calcium for maintaining bone health. In addition to providing strength to your bones and teeth, phosphorus is also essential for hormonal balance, digestion and excretion, protein production, and improved growth and cellular repair. Phosphorus is vital to growth, maintenance, and repair of all body tissue, including the brain. It also helps activate B vitamins and is a component of the storage form of energy in the body. A deficiency of phosphorus is very rare, but absorption can be reduced by the long-term and excessive use of antacids containing aluminum hydroxide. Phosphorus can be found in nuts and seeds, meat, eggs, fish, whole grains, wheat, and potatoes. Adults are encouraged to eat 1,000 milligrams of phosphorus a day.

LEARN TO LOVE LABELS

In the United States, the Food and Nutrition Board of the National Academies of Sciences, Engineering, and Medicine is responsible for establishing and updating nutrition guidelines. The recommended dietary allowances (RDAs) they establish have been the benchmark for adequate nutritional intake in the United States since the early 1940s. The RDAs are based on scientific evidence. They reflect the amount of a nutrient that is sufficient to meet the requirement of 97 to 98 percent of healthy individuals in a particular life stage and gender group. To ensure that you're getting adequate amounts of brain-nourishing vitamins like vitamin C, check the nutrition labels on food you purchase. You may be surprised at how little—or how much—various foods contribute to your RDA of brain-boosting vitamins.

SOW YOUR WILD OATS

Studies have shown that foods that are high in soluble fiber, such as oatmeal, may help to lower LDL (bad) cholesterol without lowering HDL (good) cholesterol. Oatmeal is also an important source of glucose, which is what powers your brain. Recently, researchers at the University of South Australia found out that oats can hold off cognitive decline. That's a good reason to eat oatmeal. Oat bran, which is bran that is removed from the whole oat, has similar benefits to oatmeal. You'll find oat bran in the cereal aisle of the supermarket, alongside the oatmeal, and in health food stores. Try sprinkling oat bran on cereal and yogurt. Add it to toppings for fruit crisps and casseroles. Use it to coat chicken, lean meat, or fish before baking. Mix it into meatloaf or meatballs in place of some of the bread crumbs.

Whether you choose steel-cut oats (the most roughly cut and least processed), rolled oats (also called old-fashioned), or quick oats (also called instant), all three types of oats are effective at reducing cholesterol. To get your recommended daily 3 grams of soluble fiber, you'll need to eat 2 ounces of oat bran ($^2/_3$ cup dry or about $1^1/_2$ cups cooked) or 3 ounces of oatmeal (1 cup dry or 2 cups cooked).

LET IT ALL HANG OUT

Feelings and emotions are almost identical in context. However, there are subtle differences. A feeling is a bodily sensation. If you stub your toe, you feel pain. Emotions are involuntary physical responses to events in life. A blush, a laugh, an increased heart rate, and tears are all examples of emotional reactions. An emotion may be fleeting or it may remain for days, or even years. The ability to feel enables a person to identify an emotion as something that is either positive or negative. It is when an individual represses an undesirable emotion (such as hidden anger, guilt, or self-hatred) that psychological damage can occur. It is extremely stressful to keep the lid on emotions. Acknowledging your emotions and working your way through them will free up your brain for healthier pursuits.

EAT YOUR (SEA) VEGGIES

Gram for gram, sea vegetables are higher in essential vitamins and minerals than any other known food group. They're also an important source of iodine; if your iodine level is too low, you may suffer from brain fog, memory loss, and depression. The following is a descriptive list of what sea vegetables can add to your daily diet:

- Sea vegetables can contain as much as 48 percent protein.
- Sea vegetables are a rich source of both soluble and insoluble dietary fiber.
- Sea vegetables contain significant amounts of vitamin A, in the form of beta-carotene, as well as the B complex vitamins, and vitamins C and E.
- Sea vegetables are high in potassium, calcium, sodium, iron, and chloride.
- Sea vegetables provide the fifty-six minerals and trace minerals that your body requires to function properly.

Dried sea vegetables are readily available throughout the country. Fresh sea vegetables are easier to find near the coasts. Commonly available sea vegetables are dulse and nori. Arame and wakame have mild flavors and are a good place to start.

GET AWAY FROM IT ALL

Nothing stimulates the mind quite like the experiences you have when you visit a new country. You're seeing new sights, eating new food, and listening to a different language. Travel engages the parts of your brain that are involved in creativity, and it gets the neurons firing. Sometimes our home environment is the biggest stressor in our lives. Getting away from it for a while can help you relax and gain some perspective.

A study in the *Journal of Personality and Social Psychology* found that students who studied abroad were more open to new experiences. You don't have to travel to the other side of the world. But you should make an effort to engage with a culture that isn't yours, one that is new and exciting. You'll be glad you did! If money is a worry, make it a low-cost holiday, perhaps one of those vacations where you volunteer to build a house or teach a class. Most important, don't take your problems with you! Leave work at the office and home problems at the front door. Give your brain, your body, and your soul a break.

HAVE AN ORGASM

Sex not only feels good, it's good for you. Regular sexual activity is good for your brain, mood, and memory, and it also assists with pain relief. Having sex three times a week decreases risk of stroke by 50 percent. Regular sexual activity ultimately can help you live longer. This isn't just theory—it's clinical fact. A Duke University longitudinal study on aging found a strong correlation between the frequency and enjoyment of sexual intercourse and longevity.

Sex itself is great and orgasms are even better. During orgasm, blood flows into the right prefrontal cortex, creating that fabulous sense of release and gratification. Orgasms also stimulate deep emotional parts of the brain and thus provide a calming influence. Those who have orgasms experience less depression than those who do not. According to Werner Habermehl, a German sex researcher, the more sex you have, the smarter you become. He credits the stimulation of adrenaline and cortisol during lovemaking, plus the bonus surge of serotonin and endorphins that follows orgasm. Regular orgasms ultimately lead to a boost in self-esteem.

CHARGE UP WITH GRAPE JUICE

Want to supercharge your neurons? Or at least have a better shot at remembering where you put your car keys? Drink some grape juice. In one study conducted at the University of Leeds, "highly stressed" subjects (working women between forty and fifty years old with preteen children) who drank about 12 ounces of grape juice showed immediate improvement in brain performance. Some of the gains continued even after the subjects stopped drinking the juice. An earlier study showed that a group of older adults with mild cognitive decline had improvements in memory after drinking somewhat more grape juice. There is also some evidence that drinking grape juice can lower blood sugar levels, helping protect against diabetes, which is associated with dementia (although the diabetes-dementia connection is not entirely clear to researchers). The polyphenols in grape juice are antioxidants and help rid your brain of pesky free radicals.

GET SOME GINSENG

Ginseng, one of the most popular herbal remedies in the world, is thought to aid brain function by improving memory and learning. In one study, reaction time, attention, and discrimination (responding appropriately to different situations) were all positively affected in people who took ginseng supplements. A study reported in 2017 showed that the use of ginseng helped prevent stress-related depression and anxiety by affecting the brain's hormonal response to stress. The active chemicals in ginseng, called ginsenosides, are known to help support nerve growth and neurotransmission. This, in turn, helps protect the brain during times of acute (sudden) stress. Different kinds of ginseng exist, but much of the research is focused on Korean red ginseng. A standard dose is 200 milligrams daily, and a standard extract has 4 to 7 percent ginsenosides. Check the label before using.

GET A GOOD RUB

It may feel like an indulgence, but getting a good back rub is actually a smart investment in your brain. Studies show that after a massage, people were more alert and able to solve problems faster—in some cases, twice as fast! Massage also helps you relax and get a good night's sleep, which is critical in maintaining brain health. A recent meta-analysis of the literature shows that massage therapy can keep depression at bay, and several other studies support the idea that massage can reduce anxiety. It is well known that massage helps lift your mood. It stimulates your brain to release dopamine and oxytocin, two of the feel-good brain drugs your body produces to help stabilize mood. At the same time, massage seems to dampen the production of cortisol—the stress hormone. Some research shows that the part of your brain associated with feeling happy is more active during a massage.

In general, a shorter rub helps sharpen your attention. If you need to be on your A game, a fifteen-minute back rub might be just the ticket. A longer, slower massage is more suited to helping you relax and ward off insomnia. It takes about fifteen minutes of rubbing for the feel-good drugs to start percolating in your brain. And while a one-time massage provides you with positive effects, the benefits are cumulative. This means the more you do it, the better it is for your brain. This is particularly true of the mood-enhancing benefits of massage—it is easier to maintain your positive state of mind if you get a regular massage.

PLAY CHESS

Playing chess can actually increase your IQ level. Various studies over the years have shown that young people who play chess show significant intelligence gains, including increased verbal and math skills. These benefits are earned by playing the game a few hours a week over the course of several months. Researchers theorize that the level and concentration needed to play the game stimulates the brain. While the IQ-boosting effect is most pronounced in children from grade school through high school, older players also show benefits. A study of grand master chess players showed they had enhanced activity in their frontal and parietal lobes, areas associated with problem-solving and pattern recognition. Researchers also found that playing chess used both sides of the brain. Activities that stimulate both sides of the brain are known to help strengthen the whole brain. Another study showed that older people (over age seventy-five) who played chess had less likelihood of developing Alzheimer's.

HYPNOTIZE YOURSELF

Hypnosis isn't just about getting a grown man to quack like a duck. It can also be used to decrease stress and improve cognition. Hypnosis is basically a type of meditation that can induce the theta state in your brain—a state of relaxed brain activity that is comparable to REM sleep. You may remember that REM sleep is crucial to the health of your body and that it is the point in the sleep cycle where you dream. Researchers say that achieving this state helps you relax, improves your creativity, increases mental clarity, and improves cognitive performance.

While you can be hypnotized by someone else or by listening to guided hypnosis audio programs, you can hypnotize yourself by following a few simple steps. First, find a quiet space where you can be alone. Make sure you're comfortable—that your clothing is nonrestrictive and you're in a comfortable position. Try sitting instead of lying down, because you don't want to fall asleep! Then focus on an image—a relaxing picture of a sunset, a candle flame—and take a few deep breaths. Say a positive affirmation, something like, "I am relaxed and calm." Keep repeating this affirmation while you focus on the image and continue taking deep, relaxing breaths. After a few repetitions, stop saying the affirmation but continue breathing deeply and focusing on the image. Stay in this relaxed state for ten or fifteen minutes (or longer if you'd like). Then bring yourself out of it by saying something to connect you to the real world: "I am now awake, refreshed, and ready." Then do a few simple exercises, like stretching or touching your toes, to bring you back to your usual waking state.

KNIT ONE, PURL ONE

Crafts like knitting and crocheting can improve your brain health by helping you relax. According to Herbert Benson, MD, author of *The Relaxation Response*, the rhythmic and repetitive nature of knitting can put your brain in a meditative state. It requires you to pay attention but, once you're past the learning stage, doesn't create stress (unless you've just discovered you dropped a stitch five rows back). This type of relaxed awareness benefits your brain significantly. Knitting and similar crafts actually reduce the amount of cortisol, a stress hormone, in your brain. While you're knitting, your brain is less likely to ruminate and focus on negative or depressing thoughts, which may be one reason why knitting is linked with improved mood. By the same token, it can help distract you from anxious thoughts.

A recent study published in the *Journal of Neuropsychiatry and Clinical Neurosciences* showed that older adults who knitted or crocheted were less likely to develop memory problems and suffer cognitive decline as compared to adults who read newspapers and magazines. One researcher speculates that knitting stimulates the creation of neural pathways, which helps prevent cognitive decline. Some evidence suggests that knitting can even have a therapeutic effect for people with diseases like Parkinson's, since the entire brain is used in the process. Getting all parts of the brain working together improves brain function. Knitting may also stimulate your ability to think creatively and to remember. Following complex directions can also help boost mental skills. In addition to all the brain benefits, you can produce hats, scarves, and mittens to share with friends and family!

LOAD UP ON CAROTENOIDS

Carotenoids, the compounds that give orange and yellow foods like carrots their color, aren't just bright pigments that make the garden pretty. They're also nutritional powerhouses that help keep your brain sharp. In addition to being antioxidants and playing an instrumental role in preventing heart disease and certain forms of cancer, carotenoids enhance brain function. One study showed that people with low levels of certain types of carotenoids fared badly on tests of mental function, including mental quickness, memory, and recognition.

It has been well established that one carotenoid, lutein, is important to eye health, but recent research shows that it is crucial for brain health as well. Although lutein makes up only about 12 percent of the carotenoids people eat, it makes up about 60 percent of the carotenoids in the brain, meaning the brain specifically "prefers" it. In fact, some researchers have linked lower levels of lutein in the brain with cognitive decline. Other researchers are studying the possibility that the consumption of carotenoids may prevent or delay Alzheimer's.

Your body can't produce carotenoids on its own, so you have to eat them in your diet. They can be found in abundance in carrots, broccoli, cantaloupe, cauliflower, green leafy vegetables (such as kale and spinach), and tomatoes. Some research suggests that it is easier for the body to access the carotenoids in these plants if they are cooked first to help break down the cell walls, so don't rely only on fresh salads—also cook these foods in soups and stir-fries to bring out their best nutritional value.

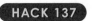

HANG OUT WITH A SMART PERSON

One of the best ways to spark up your brain is to have an intellectually stimulating conversation. Trying to wrap your mind around new ideas and concepts forces your brain to wake up and pay attention. By surrounding yourself with smart people who can challenge your thinking, you'll improve your cognition and memory. Having a debate with a friend isn't just socializing—although socializing is also good for your brain—it forces you to make logical connections between ideas and to do it on the fly. (Working under pressure is a great way to stimulate those little gray cells.) Plus, you'll probably learn something new.

FIXATE ON FLAVONOIDS

Though flavonoids have long been known to help prevent heart disease and blood clots, researchers now believe they also support brain health. One way they do this is by protecting the brain from neurotoxins. Some research suggests flavonoids may aid memory, learning, and overall cognitive function as well. They may help spur the growth of cells in the hippocampus, a part of the brain associated with memory. In addition, they work as antioxidants. They may also potentially protect against a variety of brain disorders, particularly age-related degeneration such as dementia, Alzheimer's, and Parkinson's. Researchers believe neuroinflammation contributes to the onset of these diseases by killing nerve cells, as well as adding to the brain injury that occurs in strokes. Flavonoids may help reduce neuroinflammation and protect against cell death. Recent studies show that flavonoids aid communication among neurons, support new cell growth, and help nerve cells adapt to changes ("synaptic plasticity").

A recently concluded long-term study showed that eating flavonoids helped healthy people do better on cognitive tests, with the improvement being cumulative—those who ate flavonoids over a long period of time performed significantly better than those who did not.

Because flavonoids help improve blood flow, they also create an indirect benefit for the brain, as cardiovascular problems such as hardening of the arteries can cause stroke. Plus, better circulation brings more nutrients to the brain.

New research suggests that flavonoids from citrus fruits have an easier time crossing the blood-brain barrier, so stock up on those oranges and limes! Other sources of flavonoids include apples, cranberries, endive, grape juice, kale, onions, and red wine.

MEET SAMe

SAMe (pronounced "Sammy") is a form of the amino acid methionine that occurs naturally in the body and is used for many essential functions, such as making cartilage. SAMe appears to increase the levels of certain neurotransmitters, and may thereby affect moods and emotions. In nine studies, SAMe compared favorably with antidepressant drugs, including imipramine, amitriptyline, and clomipramine. Some researchers have found that SAMe supplementation has improved mood disorders without the side effects of other antidepressants (such as weight gain, headaches, sleep disturbances, and sexual dysfunction). And SAMe works faster than some prescription antidepressants, often in four to ten days compared with two to six weeks for such drugs. However, when it comes to taking SAMe as a relief from psychological problems, never attempt to self-medicate—always consult your doctor. Absolutely do not take SAMe when you are already taking drugs for bipolar depression, obsessive compulsive disorder, or addictive tendencies, as it has been known to worsen symptoms.

SHARE WISDOM

To boost your brain, teach a continuing education class. In addition to the joy that comes with sharing your life wisdom, teaching helps strengthen mental function through reading, self-learning, and lecturing. Teaching is also a great way for you to learn new things ("While we teach, we learn," said the great Roman philosopher Seneca). Plus, teaching can provide a useful social outlet and feeling of purpose. Everyone is adept at something, so choose your specialty, approach a local continuing education program, and improve the world with your knowledge. You don't need a teaching degree, just experience.

SAY IT LOUD, SAY IT PROUD

One way to improve your memory is to speak out loud. One researcher found that when people were asked to memorize a list, those who read it out loud were able to remember better than those who read it silently. Reading out loud uses the auditory pathways of the brain, not just the visual, helping the brain to remember. A study conducted by researchers at the Université de Montréal found similar results, although in that study researchers found that addressing someone else had even better memory benefits. The researchers theorize that increasing the number of "aspects" to the information (the movement of your mouth, using speech, etc.) helps you remember it. In other words, the multisensory approach helps your brain remember and recall. So if you're studying for a test or trying to remember the three things you need from the grocery store, say it out loud.

SAY YES TO BOTANICALS

Phenolic compounds ("botanical phenolics") are antioxidants. Reactive oxygen species (ROS), a type of free radical, factors into degenerative brain diseases like Parkinson's and Alzheimer's. Through various adverse effects on cells, ROS causes cell death. Foods rich in antioxidants, such as phenolic compounds, can reduce the number of free radicals, including ROS, and may help slow or prevent these diseases. Several epidemiological studies and several meta-analyses suggest that over the long term, diets with lots of phenolic compounds offer protection from degenerative brain diseases. They are also believed to protect against cancers and some cardiovascular diseases. To add them to your diet, eat plenty of fruits, vegetables, and cereal grains, and drink green or black teas.

STOP AND SMELL THE PRIMROSE

Evening primrose oil has been shown to help lower blood cholesterol, which is good for your circulatory system and thus good for your brain. Some studies have also shown that it helps enhance memory and can calm hyperactive mental states, although research regarding its usefulness in treating attention deficit hyperactivity disorder (ADHD) has been mixed. Swedish studies, though preliminary, are relating evening primrose oil to an antioxidant that counteracts the formation of free radicals, which are destructive to brain health. If you have seizures or schizophrenia and take medications to treat it or take blood thinners or blood pressure medication, check with your healthcare provider before taking primrose oil supplements.

TALK TO YOUR DOC

If you're trying to power up your brain, the last thing you need is to drain it with unintended interactions among medications and supplements you may be taking. Some medications interfere with memory and can even mimic dementia. Others are fine on their own but pose problems when taken with other medications or supplements—or even with certain kinds of food. Cardiac medications, insomnia medications, steroids, pain medications, and others can affect cognition. Talk with your doctor and pharmacist to make sure that your medications aren't hurting your brain. In some cases, a change in medication or in how you take it can make all the difference to your brain.

SUPPLEMENT WISELY

Eating a healthy and varied diet can provide the ideal mixture of vitamins, minerals, and other nutrients your brain requires. However, even people with the best intentions sometimes fall short of their nutritional needs. Today, the definition of dietary supplements covers vitamins, minerals, fiber, herbs and other botanicals, amino acids, concentrates, and extracts. The body more readily absorbs nutrients when they come from the foods we eat so, ideally, it is best to get all of your necessary nutrients from your diet. Nevertheless, some people do need assistance to receive their required daily allowances. If you're going to take a supplement to help improve your brain health, choose the product that is right for you. The following tips can help you choose a dietary supplement:

- Pick a supplement that contains at least twenty vitamins and minerals essential for good health and no more than 150 percent of the recommended dietary allowance (RDA) for each nutrient.

- Choose a supplement tailored to your needs, whether it is age, gender, or medical status.

- Check the expiration date on the bottle. Vitamins are especially perishable. After the expiration date, they are probably not very potent.

- Take the supplement only as directed on the bottle or as prescribed by your doctor.

- Keep all supplements out of the reach of children.

FLUSH OUT WITH PHYTONUTRIENTS

Phytonutrients are the vitamins and minerals derived from fruits and vegetables. They flush away toxic chemicals, help prevent free radical damage, and keep certain hormones balanced. Think of them as nature's pharmacy—free, safe, and readily available. Some key types include:

- *Allylic sulfides.* These compounds give onions, garlic, and related herbs their pungent odor and unique flavor. They raise HDL (good) cholesterol, lower blood triglyceride levels, and protect the heart. They may prevent age-related cognitive decline.

- *Indoles and isothiocyanates.* These compounds are plentiful in broccoli, cabbage, cauliflower, and mustard greens. They help stimulate enzymes known to prevent cancer and block estrogen activity in cells. They are antioxidants, and some research shows they may improve brain function.

- *Saponins.* These chemicals bind with cholesterol and help the body flush it out. They also stimulate the immune system and help prevent heart disease and certain types of cancer. They are antioxidants, so they help keep your brain healthy by getting rid of those pesky free radicals. Saponins can be found in chickpeas, nuts, oats, potatoes, soybeans, spinach, and tomatoes.

- *Lignans.* These chemicals are known antioxidants, which help support brain function by helping to eliminate free radicals. Lignans are particularly abundant in flaxseed.

- *Monoterpenes.* Yet another cancer preventative, this phytonutrient blocks the action of certain cancer-causing compounds. It is also believed to be an antioxidant that can prevent damage to neurological functions caused by free radicals. Monoterpenes can be found in citrus fruits such as oranges and grapefruit, as well as cherries.

TAKE SHORT BREAKS

When you've got a big project staring you in the face, it's tempting just to grind it out, getting up from your chair only to pour more coffee. (But who are we kidding? You've got the coffee pot sitting on your desk.) However, research shows that this single-minded focus will backfire after a while. Just as kids at school need a recess to recharge, adults at work need to take a break now and then. A recent study from the University of Illinois at Urbana-Champaign showed that taking a short break can improve your ability to focus on a task. Researchers theorize that your brain gradually loses focus when stimulated by the same thing over and over (sort of like how you learn to ignore the ticking of a clock). By giving your brain something else to chew on for a few minutes, you can return to the original task with more focus. In the study, people who interrupted a long task with brief breaks showed no loss of performance over the course of fifty minutes, while those who didn't interrupt their task did worse over time. Unlike with multitasking, where you constantly switch between tasks, deliberately taking a break is refreshing to your brain. But don't just switch from one type of task to a similar task (reading a book, then reading a blog). Instead, do something different—take a quick walk around the office, have a conversation—then get back to the original task quickly.

WATCH YOUR NERVES

All systems in the human body are vulnerable to environmental hazards such as toxic chemicals. But the nervous system, including your brain, is at special risk for some very important reasons:

- Nerve cell loss and other changes to the nervous system occur progressively during the later years of life. As a result, toxic damage may occur simultaneously with aging.
- Many neurotoxic chemicals are easily able to cross the blood-brain barrier, causing damage to sensitive regions of the brain.
- Toxic chemicals often interfere with the nervous system's sensitive electrochemical balance, inhibiting the proper communication of information throughout the body.

To help your brain out, avoid artificial sweeteners, lead (such as lead-based paints), mercury, and pesticides.

DAYDREAM

To put yourself into a state of mind that can lead to real rest, give yourself a chance to let your mind wander. This is not a meditation at all in any formal sense. To do it, sit or lie down comfortably when you can be alone and uninterrupted for an hour. Turn lights down or off and eliminate outside noises and distractions. Close your eyes and let yourself experience the silence around you. Don't try to focus on any one thought or idea—this isn't mantra meditation. Breathe in a way that's comfortable. You can consciously slow your breath down to aid in relaxation, but don't turn it into a struggle. As you do this, let your mind wander wherever it wants to go, like a puppy let outside for an airing. Follow it if you wish, see what interests it, but make no judgments. Don't push or move your mind in any particular direction. Let it go where it wants. That is the key here. So much meditation tries to harness the mind, tether it like a goat on a rope as bait for large game. Don't do that. As your mind is given the freedom to roam here and there, to play at will, it will lead you to your place of rest.

TURN DOWN THE NOISE

A recent study shows that continued exposure to loud noises permanently affects your ability to process speech. It's not just your hearing that can be affected by loud noises—it's your brain! The cumulative effect of this process may explain why older people have difficulty learning and memorizing—because their brains have greater difficulty filtering out useless stimuli, such as music or conversation. Their brains take in everything.

People who are sensitive to noise may also find their mood negatively affected by loud sounds. They are also subject to sleep problems and lower cognitive performance. Whether you have a particular sensitivity to noise or not, a little quiet helps calm you down. And by "a little" we mean a little. A recent study suggests that just two minutes of silence can confer big health benefits, mostly by helping the body relax. Another study showed that two-hour quiet periods each day helped (rat) brains grow more cells in the hippocampus, the memory center of the brain. Silence can be not only therapeutic but also remarkably energizing. Finding time each day for silence and stillness allows the body to recharge.

FLATTEN YOUR BELLY

In a study of Kaiser Permanente patients in Northern California, middle-aged people with excess visceral fat—more commonly known as belly fat—were three times more likely to suffer from dementia in their seventies and eighties than people with little to no belly fat. The researchers found these people have a much higher risk of having that visceral fat surrounding internal organs deep in their abdominal cavity. Doctors theorize that this fat may release toxins associated with atherosclerosis, or the hardening and narrowing of arteries that is frequently present in those with Alzheimer's. Researchers reported that the risk for men with belly fat goes up when his waist exceeds 40 inches; for women, it's 35 inches. Doctors recommend a combination of weight training and aerobic exercise that targets the whole body (not just the abdominals), a low-fat diet, and minimal sugar. Recent research has suggested that eating dairy products and getting plenty of sleep may help when it comes to battling belly fat.

POUR ON THE OLIVE OIL

Olives and olive oil—long an essential part of the Mediterranean diet—are high in monounsaturated fats, which can reduce "bad" cholesterol in the blood. This in turn helps reduce the likelihood of stroke. A 2017 study by researchers at Temple University showed that eating extra-virgin olive oil protects against the development of plaques and tangles characteristic of Alzheimer's. The same study also showed that olive oil supports memory and learning ability. Many nutritionists recommend the exclusive use of olive oil for fat in the diet. Olives and olive oil also contain polyphenols, which reduce oxidative stress (free radicals) in the brain. The upshot is that eating olive oil every day can help improve brain function and support memory.

CUT THE FAT

You know that a diet with the right fats helps your brain, supplying it with energy to keep going day and night. With a few simple tips, you can greatly reduce total fat, saturated fat, and cholesterol (the wrong fats) in your meals. Try the following techniques:

- Trim all visible fat from the meat before cooking.
- Use low-fat cooking methods: broil, grill, roast, braise, stew, steam, poach, stir-fry, or microwave.
- Brown meat in a nonstick skillet with little to no fat. Use a vegetable oil spray or stock to prevent sticking.
- When grilling, broiling, or roasting meat and poultry, use a rack for the fat to drip through.
- Use marinades that have little to no fat: light teriyaki sauce, orange juice, lime juice, lemon juice, tomato juice, defatted broth, or low-fat yogurt. Add fresh herbs and other spices, such as garlic powder, to marinades for more flavor.
- Oven-bake fish and/or chicken instead of frying.

GET YOUR BEAUTY SLEEP

Your body, including your brain, mends and maintains itself when you sleep. During your daily doze, your brain clears out waste, builds new pathways, forms new memories (that's why you remember things better if you sleep right after studying), and helps maintain your mood. Getting enough sleep helps keep you safe. Being sleep-deprived increases the likelihood of accidents and mistakes. Fatigue also makes it hard for you to respond quickly and effectively to anything that happens, whether it's a test you have to take or a collision you have to avoid.

Prolonged fatigue prevents the mind and body from functioning at optimal levels, depresses the immune system, and wears down the entire system—physical, mental, and emotional. Deep and genuine rest is transformative in many ways. Sleep allows the brain to juggle the input of new information to produce flashes of creative insight. It's fairly common to wake from a power nap with an "aha" moment. In other words, get plenty of rest—it's good for your brain! It's helpful to first recognize that you want to sleep well (i.e., seven to nine hours of uninterrupted sleep each night). Go to sleep and wake up at the same times. Your body, especially your brain, loves regularity. If you are someone who sleeps very late on the weekends and then has trouble waking up for work on Monday, or if you sometimes stay up late and then crash the next evening, you aren't helping yourself. Instead, seek regularity in your sleeping patterns.

GET HELMET HEAD

If you fall, hit your head, and become unconscious, you are likely bruised and bleeding, even if you can't see it. We now know that if you're unconscious for more than an hour from a head injury, you have twice the risk of developing Alzheimer's as those without such a history. After the bleeding stops and the swelling goes down following head trauma, you can still have scar tissue that may be involved in the future development of Alzheimer's. Luckily, a product out there can help: the helmet. Always wear a helmet when riding a motorcycle, skateboarding, bicycling, rock climbing, playing hockey or football, or participating in any sport where you risk a fall. In a recent study, researchers found that bikers who wore helmets had a 52 percent lower risk of severe traumatic brain injury and a 44 percent lower risk of death than those not wearing helmets. Even if you think you're a champion bicyclist, horse rider, or whatever, accidents can easily happen and wearing a helmet can help keep you from scrambling your brain.

PONDER YOUR HUNGER

We all know that overeating can result in obesity, which in turn makes you vulnerable to stroke and other problems. Several researchers have concluded that cutting back on your eating can lessen the risk of Parkinson's disease and other neurological issues. One key to avoiding overeating is to know how hungry you really are.

Before eating, take note of how hungry you are. Rate it on a scale of 0 to 10. When you rate your hunger, you can make conscious decisions of how much food you should be eating. If you're really hungry, you may want a regular-size portion. If your hunger rates on the lower end of the scale, a snack-size portion may be your best bet. Awareness of what you're doing can help you avoid mindless overeating.

GET CREATIVE WITH CREATINE

Creatine is a naturally occurring chemical that supplies energy to all cells in the body. Approximately 95 percent of creatine is stored in skeletal muscle. It can be obtained from foods such as fish and meat, which is why vegetarians are likely low in creatine. Creatine plays a pivotal role in making sure your brain is fueled evenly throughout the day, and it has been shown in several trials to significantly improve both working memory (such as remembering words from a list) and intelligence tasks that require speed of processing (such as pushing a button as quickly as possible after it lights up).

To get the most out of your creatine supplement, take fenugreek with it. Fenugreek is a popular herb in Mediterranean dishes. It has been found that taking creatine with fenugreek in the form of seed extract results in significantly increased absorption and performance. This herb gives the same effect as glucose, but without the harmful side effects of sugar. Fenugreek actually balances blood sugar, which can result in a mild mood-stabilizing effect as well.

TRY SHANKHPUSHPI

The Latin name *Convolvulus pluricaulis* isn't much harder to pronounce than the common name of this perennial herb (it's also called aloe weed). All parts of the herb are thought to possess therapeutic benefits, and they are used in Indian and Chinese traditional medicine for chronic cough, sleeplessness, epilepsy, anxiety, and more. It's primarily used to help support memory. It is thought to possess antistress, antidepressant, antianxiety, antioxidant, and even analgesic properties, but not much scientific investigation has been conducted into the effectiveness of this herb as compared to other more commonly known ones. Even so, some studies have shown that it is effective in reducing stress.

WATCH YOUR SODIUM

Recently, researchers from McGill University found that sodium is an "on/off" switch for a major neurotransmitter receptor in the brain. This means that the amount of sodium in your body has a significant influence over diseases such as epilepsy and neuropathic pain.

Sodium is an essential nutrient in the body (in small amounts). In your body, sodium regulates water levels and draws water into the bloodstream, which can increase the volume of blood and as a result can increase your blood pressure. High blood pressure makes your heart work harder, and the increased force of the blood can hurt other organs like the kidneys, brain, and eyes.

Humans don't need much sodium; according to the American Heart Association adults only need about 1,500 milligrams a day. However, most Americans actually consume 3,400 milligrams of sodium per day. Most of the sodium we consume is not actually from the salt we put onto our food; it is salt that is already in the packaged and processed foods that we buy. It's important to read food labels and try to limit your sodium intake.

Eating more potassium each day can also help balance out your blood pressure and negate some of the harmful effects of too much sodium. Foods rich in potassium like bananas, beet greens, yogurt, potatoes, spinach, sweet potatoes, tomatoes, and white beans can help increase your potassium intake and fight high blood pressure.

GET CALM WITH CHAMOMILE

Who doesn't love a nice soothing cup of chamomile tea? It's one of the most popular ways people help themselves relax. Herbalists also use it to help treat anxiety and insomnia. A recent study showed that it does seem to have anxiolytic (anxiety-reducing) properties for people with generalized anxiety disorder. The warming and soothing properties of chamomile tea promote sleep, which is pretty much the best medicine for many problems you might have. One study showed that it can reduce levels of a stress hormone in the brain, and another showed that it may have anti-seizure properties. Drink a cup or two of tea during the day for relaxation, or have some at night to promote sleep. Generally speaking, chamomile is one of the safest herbs available. However, if you are allergic to ragweed or have ever suffered anaphylactic shock, avoid this herb.

TRAIN YOUR MEMORY

Research has proved that when it comes to maintaining and strengthening your mental abilities, practice makes perfect. In one study, scientists recorded the number of words people could recall after listening to a lengthy list of random words. Before they received memory training, the older members of the study group were able to recall fewer words than the younger members. But after just a handful of memory training sessions, which included tips such as placing words in meaningful groups rather than trying to memorize them out of context, the older participants were able to triple their word recall. In another study involving children, memorization training revealed an improvement in cognitive abilities not related to the memorization training and a leap in IQ test scores of 8 percent, as reported in the *Journal of the American Academy of Child and Adolescent Psychiatry*.

People with strong memories tend to have memory centers that communicate with the visual and spatial areas of the brain. While they may not have bigger memory centers than the next person, their brain communicates with itself more efficiently. That's a result of how memory training works: you link what you're trying to remember to a visual plan. For example, to remember a series of cards, you might imagine yourself walking through a palace and seeing one diamond chandelier in the entry with three club chairs arranged on a heart-shaped rug with four corners. When it comes time to remember the sequence, you "walk" through the room and come up with a 1 (ace) of diamonds, a 3 of clubs, and a 4 of hearts. Try it! You'll soon find you have a much easier time remembering even complex information.

BE A MATH WHIZ

Improve your mathematic abilities by doing calculations in your head whenever possible. For example, balance your checkbook without the aid of a calculator. Mentally figure out sales tax on a purchase. Determine the price per ounce or unit at the grocery store. Calculate how much change you should get back whenever you hand over money. Come up with the correct tip at a restaurant without using a tip guide. Find ways to use math in your daily life. Reliance on technology tends to dull our math skills, so put your calculator app away and use your brain. If you really want to challenge your brain, study advanced mathematics or chemistry.

MORE SOY, PLEASE!

Tofu, anyone? According to experts, soy protein appears to help lower blood cholesterol levels, decrease blood clots and platelet "clumping" or aggregation (both of which can increase the risk for a heart attack or stroke), improve the elasticity of arteries (which makes blood flow better), and reduce oxidation of LDL or "bad" cholesterol, which can lower the risk of plaque formation. All of this is good news for your brain because it means eating soy can help lower your risk for stroke. Good sources of soy include defatted soy flour, isolated soy protein, miso, firm and regular tofu, soy cheese, soymilk, and soy veggie burgers. Adding one serving a day can make a difference. If you're concerned about reports linking soy to increased estrogen and potentially impairing male fertility or increasing the risk of breast cancer, the most current research says that consuming soy, even by breast cancer patients, is safe and beneficial. If you're still concerned, just remember—everything in moderation!

HAWTHORN FOR HEALTH

Your brain functions best when the body carrying it around is healthy. Hawthorn berries have been scientifically proven to lower high blood pressure, a prime risk factor for heart disease. It's also an excellent antioxidant that eliminates free radicals, the dangerous agents that roam the body and can cause damage to blood vessels, leading to atherosclerosis. Hawthorn also contains rutin, a substance that reduces the formation of plaque, a buildup of which can block blood flow and possibly lead to stroke or a heart attack. One study showed that hawthorn may provide protection for nerve cells and may reduce inflammation of brain neurons. A very preliminary finding showed hawthorn as effective in helping prevent injury from stroke. This means hawthorn shows promise in treating, if not preventing, stroke.

DO DARK CHOCOLATE!

According to study results published in the American Chemical Society's *Journal of Agricultural and Food Chemistry*, cocoa powder has nearly twice the antioxidants of red wine and up to three times the amount found in green tea. The standard for evaluating the antioxidant properties of foods is called the oxygen radical absorbance capacity (ORAC) score. Based on the US Department of Agriculture/American Chemical Society's findings, dark chocolate tested the highest for antioxidants over other fruits and vegetables. Dark chocolate came in with an ORAC score of 13,120; its closest competitor, milk chocolate, had a score of 6,740; and third was prunes at 5,770.

Dark chocolate may help lower blood pressure in people with hypertension, and has been shown to decrease levels of LDL, the "bad" cholesterol, by 10 percent. Including dark chocolate in your diet may benefit your heart by helping to block arterial damage caused by free radicals; and it may inhibit platelet aggregation, which could cause a heart attack or stroke. There have also been studies indicating that the flavonoids in cocoa relax the blood vessels, which inhibits an enzyme that causes inflammation.

RELISH SOME AVOCADOS

Avocados are a gold mine of nutrients that boost your brain health—not to mention help you maintain a healthy body. They contain a monounsaturated fat known as oleic acid, which has been shown to help lower cholesterol and prevent heart disease and arteriosclerosis. For your brain, that means a slimmer chance of stroke. Avocados are also rich in magnesium and potassium, which help to regulate blood pressure and prevent circulatory diseases such as stroke and heart disease. One cup of avocado contains 23 percent of the daily value for folate, which when combined with the monounsaturated fats plus potassium decreases your chances of cardiovascular disease and stroke. Ounce for ounce, avocados provide more magnesium than the twenty most commonly eaten fruits. They contain no starch and very little sugar, yet they provide an excellent source of usable food energy. However, one whole California avocado has about 300 calories and 35 grams of fat, 8.5 grams being monounsaturated fat. Eat small amounts of avocado for the optimum benefit.

COMMIT

When you choose a partner and commit to a mutually rewarding intimate relationship, your brain produces the hormone oxytocin, known as "the bonding hormone." Oxytocin is associated with social behavior such as trust and empathy. High levels of oxytocin support memory and help relieve stress and cognitive problems related to stress. Oxytocin is also known to influence "prosocial" behavior—that is, things like cooperation and caregiving.

Women have higher levels of oxytocin, which may improve their ability to choose one partner (and also helps them bond with their newborns), while men's levels increase fivefold following orgasm. So commit to (and have sex with!) someone for optimum brain health.

IT'S ALL ABOUT THE MODERATION

Balance and moderation are key for a healthy and optimally functioning brain. Humans have a tendency to want more of what we like. If we drink one cup of coffee in the morning and it makes us feel more alert and focused, we drink ten. Then we wonder why we can't focus! The same thing happens with everything from cake to sex. Or we go to the opposite extreme and banish all the little pleasures from our lives. We think since sugar is unhealthy, we should never have any more of it ever, and suddenly our entire life has turned into a dreary battle against high-fructose corn syrup. You can still be healthy and eat your brownies, just as long as you don't eat too many of them. With moderation as your guide, creating a lifestyle and nutritional regimen that nourishes the brain can be more enjoyable and pleasurable than you may have imagined.

GET A HOBBY

Scientists suggest that many hobbies can help stimulate our minds and stave off Alzheimer's and dementia as we get older. There's probably something in your life you feel passionate about. Maybe it's bicycling, maybe it's painting, maybe it's creating scrapbooks or doing jigsaw puzzles. That's the basis of your hobby—something that engages the creative centers of your brain. Hobbies help make neural connections between different parts of your brain. For instance, learning to play a musical instrument early in life seems to help children with the ability to do mathematics. Learning new words to beat your friends at Scrabble can build brain cells in the language centers of your brain. So think of something you really enjoy doing and make that your hobby.

PURSUE SOME TRIVIA

Trivia games can be marvelous ways to see how good you are at jogging your memory. When you're digging around in those dusty corners of your mind for the answer, your brain synapses will be firing as they ruffle through your mental files. It's even fair to buy a trivia game, read all the answer cards, and then test how good you are at remembering something freshly learned. Read the cards often and play against yourself to see how much you improve.

While the memory training aspect is helpful, the real benefit of playing trivia games, according to a recent study, is that they provide a dopamine boost when you win—without the negative side effects of, say, gambling. A round or two of trivia can improve your mood and your attitude.

LOUNGE IN A LAVENDER BATH

We all know how it is after a stressful day. Your stomach is in knots, you feel exhausted, and your brain is still racing like an overheated engine. You're super stressed. And stress, as we've said before, is very bad for brain health—for the health of your whole body, in fact. A warm, lavender-scented bath is a great way to unwind and relax your brain. It also promotes restful sleep. Lavender oil in a hot bath before bed and lavender oil on your pillow can be very relaxing. One study showed that smelling lavender oil decreased heart rate and blood pressure, making people feel more relaxed. Subjects also noted improved moods after smelling lavender oil.

PLAY WITH A PET

Stressed? Fling a Frisbee with Fido. One of the most consistent findings among the many studies evaluating the beneficial role of pets in our lives is that they provide an important measure of stress relief. Simply petting or playing with your favorite pet, whether it's a dog, cat, hamster, or canary, stimulates the production of calming chemicals within the brain and helps you relax. Watching fish in an aquarium has a similar calming effect. The calming influence of small animals is so effective that many doctors recommend daily pet play as therapy for their patients who are under a lot of stress either at work or at home. Fifteen minutes of tossing a yarn ball to some frolicsome kittens is a wonderful and inexpensive way to shed the stress of a hard day at the office. Spend time with your pet, whatever the species, and enjoy its company. Talk to it. Pet it. Scratch it behind the ears. Bask in the glow of the pet-owner bond and feel the anxiety melt away. Even the most stressful day is no match for a puppy that's so happy to see you that its tail is a blur.

PRACTICE TAI CHI

Although tai chi is technically an ancient Chinese martial art, in practice it is more art than martial. In tai chi, you perform a series of flowing, slow movements linked with specific breathing patterns. Since it doesn't create a lot of stress on the joints, and the movements can be modified, it's a great choice for individuals with physical challenges, who are older, or who need a gentler introduction to exercise than the local gym's turbo kickboxing class.

Recently, researchers from the University of South Florida and Fudan University in Shanghai studied people who practiced tai chi three times a week. They found that their brains increased in size, compared to those who didn't. Further, people who practiced tai chi did better on memory and learning tests.

Research on tai chi has found it to be helpful for mood disorders, such as anxiety and depression, as well as for physical ailments, such as arthritis and hypertension (high blood pressure). Tai chi is great for balance training, flexibility, and relaxation. Because you must learn a series of complex physical movements, practicing tai chi helps keep your brain flexible. For a low-impact exercise, tai chi has a high impact on the brain.

WORK YOUR BRAIN

As we age, we often experience difficulty understanding complex arguments, completing math problems, and figuring out visual-spatial puzzles. While sometimes these issues are a sign of early dementia, more often they are simply the result of mental inactivity—that is, people who experience these problems haven't been exercising their brain in these particular areas. Maintaining mental acuity is like training to be a professional athlete; you must pursue it vigorously. The future results are too important for this to be a half-hearted venture. The key is training and practice. You must treat your brain like a muscle, giving it a workout on a regular basis. Instead of picking a by-the-numbers murder mystery, read a more complex philosophical tome. Use a map instead of GPS. Troubleshoot your computer's error message yourself instead of hiring someone else to fix it. Your brain may complain but you'll be glad you did the heavy mental lifting.

COMBAT MIGRAINES

If you're prone to migraines, here's more bad news: migraines have been shown to have long-term effects on the structure of the brain. One of the unhappy changes is that your brain creates pathways that make it easier for you to feel pain (thanks, brain!). Other research shows that lesions on the brain are associated with migraines. To avoid these downsides, you'll want to get those migraines under control. Be sure to talk with your doctor about the best treatment plan for you and try to identify potential triggers, such as allergies and stress, so that you can do your best to avoid them.

In addition, here are two supplements you may want to consider:

1. The University of Maryland Medical Center recommends the use of extracts of the flowering plant feverfew to treat severe headaches. Feverfew inhibits the release of two substances considered to bring on migraine attacks—serotonin from platelets and prostaglandin from white blood cells. However, it is important to note that feverfew does not actually cure a migraine—it only helps prevent or lessen it. It can take several months of regular use for feverfew to work. When using capsules or tablets, be sure to read the label carefully; some brands contain only trace amounts of the pure herb. Also, consult with your physician regarding dosage.

2. Preliminary research indicates that taking a high dose (400 milligrams) of riboflavin (vitamin B_2) every day may help prevent migraine headaches. Researchers caution that you need to make sure that your headaches are true migraines, and that it works best if you have migraines at least twice a month. Most riboflavin supplements contain no more than 100 milligrams per tablet, so you'll need a prescription to get one that contains 400 milligrams. Talk to your doctor before treating your migraines with riboflavin supplements.

PROTECT WITH SELENIUM

Selenium, itself a very powerful antioxidant, also enhances the antioxidant capabilities of vitamin E. Selenium benefits the brain by preventing oxidation of fat. Free radicals, a by-product of oxidation, are damaging to your brain's health. Since more than half of the brain is composed of fat, preventing its oxidation helps slow age-related brain deterioration and preserves cognitive function. In other words, selenium is your new best friend.

Selenium also benefits the immune system, and some studies suggest that it improves circulation throughout the body. Because selenium levels tend to decline with age, older people should take selenium supplements in addition to adding selenium-rich foods to their diets. There is no established recommended dietary allowance (RDA) for selenium but note that selenium can become toxic if 700 micrograms (mcg) are consumed on a daily basis.

Natural sources of selenium include broccoli, cabbage, celery, cucumbers, garlic, onions, kidney, liver, chicken, whole-grain foods, seafood, and milk.

PLAY PING-PONG

Daniel G. Amen, MD, author of *Making a Good Brain Great*, is a major enthusiast of table tennis, calling it "the best brain sport ever." Amen writes, "It is highly aerobic, uses both the upper and lower body, is great for eye-hand coordination and reflexes, and causes you to use many different areas of the brain at once as you are tracking the ball, planning shots and strategies, and figuring out spins. It is like aerobic chess." He also noted that it is the second most popular organized sport in the world, and has been an Olympic sport since 1988. Pick up a paddle and give it a try.

READ

Reading anything is good for your brain, but novel reading is particularly healthy. A recent study by neuroscientists at Emory University found that reading novels improves your brain health by enhancing brain connectivity. Read as much as you can and focus on works that challenge you. The latest potboiler may be a fun read, but it's probably as mentally challenging as a Dick and Jane primer. You can give your brain a workout by reading a literary classic you've always meant to tackle or by reading a nonfiction book on a topic you're interested in but know nothing about. Read carefully, with memory and recall in mind. To help you assimilate this new information, discuss it with friends. So, to give your brain some exercise, find a comfortable chair and start reading.

JOIN A BOOK CLUB

Joining a book club provides a triple bonus for your brain. Most book clubs pick challenging books and set a specific deadline for reading them. Part of the fun is analyzing a book's structure, theme, characterizations, plot, and other concepts. Much of this may not be familiar to you, but that will make the experience more interesting and mentally challenging. Also, groups typically gather for discussions, offering you opportunities to socialize, engage in meaningful conversation, and invigorate yourself—all things your brain craves. It's also likely to help you stay contemporary and be more aware of what's going on in the world. Join a book club; it's a win-win-win situation.

WATCH YOUR LANGUAGE

Cliché is the French word for "stereotype." In English, *cliché* is used to describe phrases and expressions that have been so overused they've lost their freshness and original meaning. For example:

- Saved by the bell
- As old as the hills
- In the nick of time
- Haste makes waste

Clichés are boring and trite, and relying on clichés to communicate is lazy. Exercise your brain by challenging yourself to avoid clichés and come up with a fresh metaphor or an original expression. And maybe you'll create a new cliché that lazy people can use when they talk.

TELL A STORY ABOUT YOU

Writing your autobiography can be a very rewarding activity—you preserve your life experiences for the benefit of other family members and exercise your brain in the process. Recalling previous events requires a strong memory (which may be aided by going through photo albums, letters, etc.), and the act of writing improves visual-spatial skills. Expressive writing—that is, writing that tries to capture emotion and explain why and how things happened, such as you would do in a memoir—has been shown to help people cope with negative events. They experience fewer unwanted thoughts about these past events. Researchers speculate that writing it down helps free up the brain for other cognitive tasks. One study of college students showed that writing about their life experiences helped them gain insight (they used more so-called "insight" words than the control group), and it also improved their grade point averages.

SEIZE A SIESTA

It's true that we should get plenty of sleep at night—at least eight hours, say most doctors—but napping during the day can also benefit your brain. Taking forty winks improves memory according to several studies. When you form a memory, it's first stored in the hippocampus, but while it's there you can easily lose it. Napping apparently pushes memories to the neocortex, where they become more permanent.

Studies have also found that people who nap regularly have an easier time learning. Research suggests that the right hemisphere of the brain is more active during sleep, while the left side relaxes and takes some time off. After you wake up, the left side will be refreshed and ready to learn new stuff. So don't be afraid to put your feet up, close your eyes, and doze off for a while.

MAKE SOME COCOA

A nice warm cup of cocoa isn't only for warming up on a winter day. It benefits your brain. In a study done by Salk Institute for Biological Studies researcher Henriette van Praag and colleagues, a compound found in cocoa, epicatechin, combined with exercise, was found to promote functional changes in a part of the brain involved in the formation of learning and memory. Epicatechin is a flavonol, a group of chemicals that have previously been shown to improve cardiovascular function and increase blood flow to the brain (helping bring nutrition to your gray matter and helping prevent strokes). A recent study by Italian researchers found that among a group of sixty-one-year-olds to eighty-five-year-olds, those who consistently consumed cocoa tested better for attention and memory.

DON'T BE A WORRYWART

You know that worrying doesn't solve anything, but it's still an easy habit to fall into. Excessive, habitual worrying keeps your brain running around in circles. Often this puts you in fight-or-flight mode, which stresses your entire body—particularly your brain. Nearly 20 percent of adults struggle with anxiety disorders—what might be called worrying run amok. Chronic worrying can contribute to the development of psychiatric problems. When you worry, your brain produces more cortisol, a stress hormone, which can destroy brain cells and create memory and learning problems. But you can train your brain to think positively. Cognitive therapy emphasizes using positive thoughts to help you change your emotions. This helps the rational part of your brain (the cortex) get control over the irrational part (the limbic system). If you can think before you feel (or at least learn to think faster after you feel), you can reduce the amount of worry you experience. Going worry-free benefits your brain!

GO PUBLIC

Cutting down on TV watching in general is a good way to take care of your brain. If you're going to watch, though, PBS offers intelligent programming that will inform, educate, and stimulate your brain. Forgo the mindless and mind-numbing shows that commercial stations fill the airwaves with. In the same way we become what we think (or eat), we also become what we watch. Don't clutter your brain with the equivalent of junk food. Pick and choose carefully, and select shows that involve or educate your brain. Doing so will not only make you mentally sharp, but it will also liven up your conversation when socializing.

TAKE RESPONSIBILITY

Modern healthcare encourages people to rely on others to make decisions for them. Experts tell us what to do. Relief from our medical problems is just a prescription away. While it's natural to turn to experts and to accept help, be sure you're not also giving up responsibility for your own health. It's up to you to make good decisions about how to live your life, what to eat and how much, what to drink and how much, how you work and how you play. Although you might be able to banish the results of an unhealthy choice by taking a little colored pill, it's better to step back and think about the choices you're making. Develop an awareness of your life's complexity—your body, mind, emotions, and spirit—and how these elements interact. Use others to get the information to make the right decisions—but in the end, it's up to you to take responsibility to know what is and isn't good for your brain.

PROTECT YOUR HEARING

Noise isn't just an irritation, it can hurt your brain. While aging does take its toll on your ability to hear, noise itself is the other big culprit. The greater your exposure to noise, the greater the likelihood that you'll suffer hearing impairment. In the bad news category, researchers at Johns Hopkins University found that people with hearing impairments were 30 to 40 percent more likely to experience cognitive decline. People with hearing loss appear to lose brain mass at a greater rate than those who have good hearing. Hearing loss also increases the demand on the brain because of the effort involved when a person with hearing loss tries to hear and process what is being said. This can add to stress too. It isn't clear whether the use of hearing aids can help reverse the likelihood of dementia. What is clear, though, is you should protect those precious ears! Noise levels over 105 decibels can damage your ears if you're exposed to them for more than fifteen minutes per week. Levels over 80 decibels can damage your hearing if you are frequently exposed to them (for several hours per day). A forklift runs at about 90 decibels, so just working in a warehouse could damage your hearing if you don't use ear protection. Some simple ways to save your hearing:

- Use earplugs or ear protection in noisy environments.
- Turn it down—listen to music, the television, and so on, at lower volumes.
- Give your ears a break—silence can help your hearing recover. Without it you risk permanent damage.

CLOSE YOUR EYES

Your brain relies on your vision to make sense of the world. But given the complicated way your brain perceives visual images, it's basically just hallucinating what it thinks is there, based on incomplete information. It's no small wonder it gets things wrong from time to time. One researcher found that blindfolding participants enhanced their other senses. Subjects quickly learned to navigate unfamiliar terrain even without the help of vision by listening, smelling, and touching. A different study showed that sitting quietly with a blindfold for just ninety minutes improved participants' hearing. Other research suggests that doing tasks while blindfolded can improve memory, motor skills, and problem-solving. Should you break out a blindfold and try to make dinner? Probably not. But closing your eyes and letting other senses do some work may stimulate your brain.

THINK HOLISTICALLY

Even though we've been talking about the brain by itself, you can't think of it as existing in isolation. It's bound up with the rest of you—your lungs, liver, spleen, bones, blood—the whole you. Each part of your body works in concert with all the other bits. The brain is one of the most important organs you have, but it's not the only one. To make your brain healthier, think of yourself holistically. As the musician Mick Fleetwood said, "I keep fit, I work out, I eat pretty damn well, I don't drink like a fish, and all of those things are tempered with a holistic mind-set that you need to damn well respect the vehicle that you're walking around in."

Exactly!

OPEN A WINDOW

Make sure your home is well ventilated. Open all the windows whenever possible and consider exhaust fans or air-to-air heat-exchanging devices that draw in fresh air through one duct and expel it through another. In addition, make sure stoves and heaters all vent outdoors. Keeping your house constantly closed tight not only prevents harmful pollutants from dissipating, but it also promotes sick building syndrome, a condition in which occupants suffer adverse health effects seemingly related to conditions in their living space. Sick building syndrome can include brain-defeating symptoms like dizziness, fatigue, and difficulty concentrating. At work, try to encourage coworkers to keep windows open. If that's not possible—many office buildings have windows that don't open—at least take breaks throughout the day and go outside for a breath of fresh air.

ADD DIVERSITY TO YOUR SOCIAL LIFE

According to researchers, the more people participate in close social relationships, the better their overall physical and mental health, and the higher their level of function. The definition of *social relationship* is broad and can include everything from daily phone chats with family and regular visits with close friends to attending church every Sunday. The MacArthur Foundation Research Network on an Aging Society revealed that the two strongest predictors of well-being among the elderly are frequency of visits with friends and frequency of attendance at organization meetings. The more meaningful the contribution in a particular activity, the greater the health benefit. And these interactions shouldn't always be with people who believe what you believe. Studies show that the more diverse your innermost circle of social support, the better off you are. Recent psychological research says that because the brain is inherently lazy (that's why it likes to rely on stereotypes in the first place), challenging it with diversity actually helps keep it running in tip-top shape.

PAY ATTENTION!

Many of us stumble through life paying attention only to what we absolutely have to and marginally noticing everything else. This low ability to focus creates problems in organizing and remembering information and makes it difficult to finish tasks. Focusing intently on a particular project, new skill, or task hones your brain's ability to absorb, order, and retain information. Paying close attention, really focusing, essentially keeps your brain sharp and pliable. But what is focus?

Your brain has three types of focus, which researchers call attention:

1. Selective attention, which you use when you're doing one task and filtering out other input—filing your nails is an example of selective attention.

2. Divided attention, which you use when you have to pay attention to several sources of input—crossing a street is a good example. You have to pay attention to where you're walking and look out for cars at the same time (in reality your brain switches between these tasks).

3. Focused attention, which you use when you concentrate on one task for a long time—writing a lengthy report without interruption, for example.

Focused attention is the type of focus that most people mean when they talk about having trouble focusing. But the fact is, researchers say people actually struggle more with tasks that require divided attention because it is more tiring for the brain. Research shows that the best way to build all of these types of focus is through practice—so practice crossing the street, filing your nails, and writing that report without getting distracted by *Facebook*, the television show you'd rather be watching, or your neighbor's yappy dog.

EXPERIMENT WITH ESSENTIAL OILS

Essential oils are distillations of plants that have plant-specific beneficial properties. Using the calming essential oils can help your brain by banishing stress. Some of the most popular include lavender, sage, sandalwood, frankincense, and chamomile. You can light scented candles, place fragrant potpourri throughout your home, or put a few drops of scented oil in your bathwater or on your pillow. Floral scents tend to work best, because food scents can make you hungry. Avoid tart or biting fragrances, such as lemon, because they may have the opposite effect, perking you up instead of calming you down. You may have to experiment until you find the scent that is right for you.

Don't use essential oils under the following conditions without the consultation of a qualified practitioner:

- If you are pregnant
- If you have allergies
- If you are receiving medical or psychiatric treatment
- If you are taking homeopathic remedies
- If you have any chronic or serious health problems, such as a heart condition

However, aromatherapy is safe to use at home for minor or short-term problems, such as mild depression or tension, so long as you follow safety guidelines:

- Do not take essential oils internally or put them in your eyes.
- Do not use essential oils to treat young children.
- Keep all oils away from children.
- Do not apply undiluted oils directly to the skin.

FLIRT

According to Daniel G. Amen, MD, author of *Making a Good Brain Great*, when you feel an attraction to someone, areas deep in the brain, which are rich in the neurotransmitter dopamine, light up with pleasure. Extra dopamine courses through your body and brain, generating feelings of well-being. Your brain stem also activates, releasing phenylethylamine (PEA), which speeds the flow of information between nerve cells. "Taken together, the release of dopamine and PEA explains why, when we are around someone we are attracted to, we feel a 'rush' and our hearts beat faster. Attraction is a powerful drug," reports Dr. Amen.

What does this have to do with flirting? Well, you flirt with people you're attracted to (and hopefully they flirt back). The beauty of flirting is that there's little risk to it. If you make an initial conversation starter and it's not reciprocated, no big deal. But if your flirting is reciprocated, that lights up the pleasure centers of your brain and encourages you to do more, which gives you more dopamine, and the next thing you know, you're a very happy person. So, add a little flirting to your life. It's good for your brain.

GET OUT IN THE SUN

Everyone knows that going out in the sun without sunscreen is bad, bad, bad. Right? Not so fast. "The push to prevent skin cancer may have come with unintended consequences," Diane Welland wrote in an article for *Scientific American*. See, one of the easiest ways to get vitamin D, which helps neurotransmitters work, is to let the sun shine in. But if you slather your skin with sunscreen, your body can't soak up that delicious vitamin D. People who use sunscreen all the time can create problems for their brains.

A study conducted by a group of European scientists found that subjects with vitamin D deficiency performed poorly on a number of tests. The less vitamin D they had, the worse their performance.

The body can get vitamin D from two sources—food and the sun. This vitamin is known as the "sunshine vitamin" because the body can make vitamin D after sunlight hits the skin. Your body's ability to produce vitamin D from sunlight diminishes with age; therefore, requirements increase for older adults. Foods rich in vitamin D include fortified milk or juice, salmon, tuna, mushrooms, mackerel, and fortified breakfast cereals.

Because vitamin D is a fat-soluble vitamin, it can be toxic in larger doses. Toxicity can lead to kidney stones or damage, weakened muscles and bones, excessive bleeding, and other health problems. Levels high enough to cause health complications usually come from supplements, not from food or too much sunlight. If you take a supplement that includes vitamin D, make sure it does not contain more than you need for your age range and gender. Vitamin D has a UL (upper limit) set at 50 micrograms (mcg) or 2,000 IUs (international units) per day for children and adults. There is no UL established for infants.

DON'T SKIP MEALS

You need to fuel your brain throughout the day with nutritious food. Skipping meals can have numerous negative effects on your healthy lifestyle. Going without food for too long can make you so hungry that you overeat at your next eating opportunity, and you likely won't eat as healthfully as you would have otherwise. Skipping meals can negatively affect your productivity, concentration, and energy level. Since your brain runs on glucose, not giving it enough makes you lose your ability to focus. If you go without for a long time, your brain basically stops being able to do anything but think about how hungry you are. Plus, your mood turns nasty. "Hangry" much? So make time and even schedule eating opportunities throughout the day.

TRY A BRAIN-HEALTHY DIET

It can't be overstated that what you eat affects the way your brain works. The brain gobbles up a huge proportion of the nutrients we put in our body. If those nutrients aren't what they're supposed to be, your brain will get off track.

Here are the seven parts of a daily brain-healthy diet:

1. Eat six to eleven servings of grains (bread, cereal, rice, pasta, and other grain foods). A serving is about ½ cup of oatmeal, 1 ounce uncooked pasta or rice, or one slice of bread.

2. Eat at least three servings of vegetables. A serving of vegetables is generally 1 cup; for raw leafy greens, it's 2 cups.

3. Eat at least two servings of fruit. A serving is one medium fruit, or ½ cup canned or chopped fruit.

4. Eat two or more servings of low-fat or fat-free dairy products, such as milk, yogurt, and cheese. A serving of dairy is generally 1 cup of milk or yogurt, or 1.5 ounces of cheese.

5. Eat two to three servings of lean meat, poultry, fish, dried beans, eggs, or nuts. A serving is 1 ounce lean meat, ¼ cup cooked beans, or ½ ounce nuts.

6. Eat a varied diet.

7. Eat at least three well-balanced meals each day.

If you fall short on any of these behaviors, you may benefit from taking a daily multivitamin and mineral supplement. Supplements are not meant to take the place of any food group or meal, but they can help round out what you may not eat every single day. Choose one food group at a time and try to gradually improve your daily eating pattern. Aim to eat at least the minimum number of servings each day.

BE GRATEFUL

When you focus on what you love about your life, your emotional brain fires up. Gratitude helps support mental health. Many studies show that expressing gratitude helps healthy people stay healthy and reduces their feelings of depression and anxiety. Interestingly, a recent study of people suffering from depression and anxiety showed that writing a gratitude letter helped improve their mental health. People who used negative words in their writing gained fewer mental health benefits, suggesting that it's the absence of negative words that helps people get the biggest boost from gratitude. Researchers theorize that writing about what you're grateful for moves your attention away from negative emotions like envy and anger. You're therefore less likely to fixate on bad things or experiences. The mental health benefits are true even if you don't share your gratitude with anyone. The study also suggested that the effects are cumulative, so that if you practice gratitude frequently, you'll see better results over a long time. So write out five things you're grateful for today. Focus on what is making you feel lucky and good about your life. This trains your brain to focus on the love and pleasant experiences in your life. Do it long enough and you'll effectively create a positive groove in your brain that will create ripple effects in your life.

TRACK DOWN TRACE MINERALS

Your body needs minerals such as cobalt, fluoride, and iodine to function well. Although they make up only about 4 percent of the body, minerals are crucial to good brain functioning. You get minerals only from food (your body can't make them), so you need to eat a diet rich in minerals. While it is well known that you need certain minerals such as calcium, potassium, and phosphorus—and don't forget the iron!—of the thousands of known minerals, scientists aren't completely sure how many of them are necessary for good health. That's because your body needs only trace amounts of some minerals, and not every single one of the thousands we know about have been studied for their effect on the human body.

We do know you need trace minerals like the hard-to-pronounce molybdenum. Even though the amount needed is small—most trace minerals are measured in micrograms (mcg)—they are still very important to proper health. There are no recommended dietary allowances (RDAs), dietary reference intakes (DRIs), or safe and adequate ranges set for these minerals because not enough is known about what the body requires for proper health and functioning. A healthy, varied, and balanced diet is the best way to ensure you consume safe and adequate amounts of trace minerals.

GET YOUR BLOOD FLOWING

Several recent studies have shown that vinpocetine, a health supplement that originates from the periwinkle plant, can provide a significant boost to memory and concentration. A recent study published in the *Annals of Medical and Health Sciences Research* included patients with cognitive impairment. It showed that taking a 5 milligram dose twice a day for twelve weeks was enough to improve memory and concentration. Like other highly effective brain supplements, vinpocetine is able to cross the blood-brain barrier, allowing it to directly affect the brain, leading to improved cognition. Vinpocetine is so beneficial because it acts in a few different ways. It has anti-inflammatory qualities, which can help improve the function of the mind and body, and its antioxidant properties and vasodilating effects (widening of blood vessels) are likely responsible for the improvement in cognition. Neuroimaging studies have shown an increase in cerebral blood flow, which is especially important for those that have cerebrovascular disease. Vinpocetine is available as a supplement by itself, but many companies mix vinpocetine with other compounds for an increased effect.

DANCE, DANCE, DANCE

While studying the effects of different types of exercise on the brain, researchers at the University of Illinois at Urbana-Champaign and other institutions found that the participants who danced for one-hour sessions three times a week showed an improvement in some of the white matter of their brains (namely, the fornix, the part that controls processing speed and memory), while the participants who did a walking or stretching regimen showed the white matter degeneration that is characteristic of aging. Dance has proven so effective at helping the brain that it is now being used to treat people with Parkinson's. In the past decade, researchers have become more interested in why dance is so beneficial to the brain. They theorize that music stimulates the reward centers of the brain, making you feel good and reducing stress, while the physical movements activate sensory and motor parts of the brain (among other parts). Overall, then, dance involves much of the brain, helping improve brain health as it strengthens memory and the connections between nerve cells. One study showed that of a number of physical activities such as golf and swimming only dance actually decreased the risk of dementia. So dust off your dancing shoes and hit the floor.

ZINC-IFY YOUR DNA

Zinc aids the brain as part of a metabolic process that eliminates harmful free radicals. It also strengthens neuronal membranes for greater protection and helps get rid of lead, which can enter the brain by way of automobile exhaust and other sources and adversely affect mental function. Zinc is part of the molecular structure of dozens of important enzymes. It is a component of the insulin that regulates your energy supply, and it works with red blood cells to transport waste carbon dioxide from body tissue to the lungs, where it is expelled. Zinc is also vital to the production of the RNA and DNA that oversee the division, growth, and repair of the body's cells, including brain cells. Dietary sources of zinc include beef, herring, seafood, pork, poultry, milk, soybeans, and whole grains. The recommended dietary allowance (RDA) for zinc is 15 milligrams, not to exceed 40 milligrams per day, for adults over eighteen years of age. Women who are pregnant may want to take an additional 5 milligrams of zinc daily, and women who are breastfeeding should take an extra 10 milligrams daily.

BREAK THE FAST

The word *breakfast* describes exactly what it does: breaks a fast. After a good night's rest, your body has gone eight to twelve hours without food or energy. Blood sugar, or glucose, which comes from the breakdown of food in the body, is your body's main source of energy. Eating food provides your body with a fresh supply of blood glucose or energy. The brain in particular needs a fresh supply of glucose each day because that is its main source of energy. (The brain does not store glucose.) Eating breakfast is associated with being more productive and efficient in the morning hours. Breakfast eaters tend to experience better concentration, problem-solving ability, strength, and endurance. Your muscles also rely on a fresh supply of blood glucose for physical activity throughout the day.

If you're worried that eating breakfast might make you gain weight, rest assured the opposite is true. Eating a good healthy breakfast can help regulate your appetite throughout the day. Breakfast can help you eat in moderation at lunch and dinner. Also, research indicates that a high-fiber, low-fat breakfast may make a major contribution to a total reduced fat intake for the day. If you have a hard time facing food first thing in the morning, start with eating a light breakfast, such as a piece of whole-grain toast or fruit. Then pack a breakfast or snack to take with you so you can eat once you do get hungry. Here are a few healthy suggestions:

- Cold cereal with fruit and skim milk
- Yogurt with fruit or low-fat granola cereal
- Peanut butter on a whole-wheat bagel and orange juice
- Bran muffin and a banana
- Instant oatmeal with raisins or berries
- Breakfast smoothie (blend fruit and skim milk)
- Hard-boiled egg and grapefruit juice
- Cottage cheese and peaches

RAMP UP YOUR AMINO ACIDS

Amino acids—organic compounds that help the body make proteins—are essential to human metabolism. Though amino acids don't receive nearly as much attention in nutrition discussions as vitamins and minerals, you need them just as much to stay healthy—particularly for brain function. Let's take a closer look at some of the most important amino acids in terms of maintaining mental acuity:

- *Arginine.* This amino acid is partially converted into a chemical known as spermine, which is believed to help the brain process memory. Low levels of spermine often signal age-related memory loss.

- *Choline.* The brain uses this amino acid to manufacture a memory-related neurotransmitter called acetylcholine. Older people are encouraged to take choline supplements because as we age we tend to produce less acetylcholine, putting us at greater risk of memory impairment. Dietary sources of choline include cabbage, cauliflower, eggs, peanuts, and lecithin.

- *Glutamine.* This amino acid is a precursor of a calming neurotransmitter known as GABA (gamma-aminobutyric acid). It also helps improve clarity of thought and boosts alertness by assisting in the manufacture of glutamic acid, a compound known for its ability to eliminate metabolic wastes in the brain.

- *Methionine.* Like glutamine, this amino acid helps cleanse the brain of damaging metabolic wastes. It is an effective antioxidant and helps reduce brain levels of dangerous heavy metals such as mercury.

SING!

Singing has long been connected to intelligence, creativity, emotion, and memory, according to Daniel G. Amen, author of *Making a Good Brain Great*. It has been proven that singing information or attaching a melody or jingle to it helps you retain the information. "Singing stimulates temporal lobe function, an area of the brain heavily involved in memory," Dr. Amen reports. If you can't sing, try humming, which also provides a positive difference in mood and memory. Dr. Amen says, "As the sound activates your brain, you will feel more alive and your brain will feel more tuned in to the moment."

Recent research shows that singing both calms you down and makes you feel happier, as it releases feel-good neurotransmitters. And it is known that people retain memories related to singing even when dementia has crippled other parts of the brain. Some reports suggest that people who sing frequently are more emotionally stable, have better working memory, and process information more efficiently than nonsingers. Break out the karaoke machine and boost your brain health.

CREATE

Creativity goes beyond the typical uses of the brain for thinking and gathering and assimilating information. Creativity is what happens when you relax and allow your brain to birth new thoughts, new ways of seeing, or new ways of doing. Despite all the talk about the right side of the brain being the creative side, the beauty of creativity is that it uses your whole brain. When your brain is in what researchers call the "imagination network" many regions of your brain are engaged. In addition to helping strengthen your brain, being creative is a stress-reliever. People who are considered creative tend to be happier and report greater life satisfaction. So challenge your brain by releasing it from its humdrum tasks so that it can work its imaginative magic.

DRIED BUT NOT FORGOTTEN

Fruits are loaded with many essential nutrients. Eating different fruits ensures a better intake of all the nutrients, such as trace minerals, that they provide. But sometimes keeping lots of fresh fruits on hand means that some will go bad before you get a chance to eat them. The solution? Dried fruits! These tasty treats are available all year long, and they are easy to carry with you for quick snacks when your brain and body are feeling sluggish. Try as many colors and types as you can for variety, such as prunes, figs, apricots, raisins, cherries, and mango. Just remember that because the water content has been removed, the serving size for dried fruit is roughly 75 percent of the serving size for fresh fruit, making it easy to accidentally overindulge. Always choose dried fruits with no added sugar, and look for sulfur- or sulfide-free varieties. Although the FDA has deemed small amounts of sulfur dioxide, which is used as a preservative in some dried fruits, safe to consume, those who are sensitive to it may experience breathing problems as a result.

GET SOME INCAN GOLD

Once known as "the gold of the Incas," quinoa is a complete protein that includes all nine essential amino acids, which makes it an excellent choice for anyone concerned about a healthy brain. Quinoa has extra high amounts of the amino acid lysine, which is essential for tissue growth and repair. It may also play an important role in regulating anxiety. As a whole grain, quinoa has been associated with higher levels of brain function.

Quinoa is a very good source of manganese as well as magnesium, iron, copper, phosphorus, and the B vitamins, especially folate, another essential nutrient needed for the formation and development of new and normal body tissue (your body must acquire folate from foods and supplements). Quinoa also provides riboflavin, or B_2, which is necessary for the proper production of cellular energy in your body. For such a small "grain" (it's technically a seed) quinoa provides a whole lot of nutrients.

REPEAT AFTER ME

Instead of worrying endlessly about your upcoming tax audit or dwelling on that conversation you just had with your boss, do something repetitive, such as playing solitaire or washing dishes. Not only does the distraction get your brain out of an endless negativity loop but keeping part of your brain occupied with a repetitive action actually frees up the creative side of your brain to solve problems. This is why we often have great ideas when we are in the shower or not thinking about something in particular. In addition to the possibility of creativity, repetitive action is soothing and helps reduce stress levels.

FLUSH THE TOXINS

You've probably heard of neurotoxins, those pollutants such as pesticides that can interfere with nerve function (and therefore are very bad for brain health). If you suspect that you may have been exposed to dangerous fumes or toxic chemicals, consult a doctor for a thorough analysis and treatment. To cleanse your brain (and your body) of common toxins, such as pollutants or household chemicals, you can try a variety of natural remedies. These include flaxseed, licorice root, ginseng, ginkgo biloba, aloe vera, grapefruit pectin, papayas, slippery elm bark, alfalfa, peppermint, and ginger tea. You can take capsules or use the ingredients to make tea. You can also drink lemon water, exercise strenuously, use a sauna, get a vigorous massage, and eat a high-fiber, cleansing diet. Deep breathing exercises, in clean environments, will infuse your brain with fresh oxygen. When it comes to minimizing food contaminants, wash all fruits and vegetables thoroughly.

TRY VALERIAN INSTEAD OF VALIUM

Called "the Valium of the nineteenth century" (though it has no chemical similarity to Valium), the herb valerian (*Valeriana officinalis*) is a common sedative used worldwide. In Europe, it is prescribed for anxiety. Herbalists have chosen valerian for treatment of nervous tension and even for panic attacks. It is known as a safe, non-narcotic herbal sedative and is often combined with other herbs to make pain-relieving remedies, as it has the ability to relax muscle spasms. How does valerian do its magic? Scientists believe it increases the amount of a chemical called gamma-aminobutyric acid (GABA) in the brain, which is responsible for its calming effect.

PARSLEY PARTY

Parsley is loaded with vitamin C, vitamin A, vitamin K, iodine, and iron—all nutrients your brain needs to function well. Actually, parsley has a higher vitamin C content than citrus, and thus it is an excellent ingredient to battle inflammation. Parsley is rich in flavonoids known for their antioxidant activity, meaning that it helps to prevent free radicals from damaging your body's cells. Parsley's dark green color provides oxygenating chlorophyll, which increases the antioxidant capacity of your blood. The body parts most affected by the properties in parsley are the kidneys, bladder, stomach, liver, and gall bladder, but it is also good for your brain. A recent study published in the *Journal of Nutrition* found a connection between a flavonoid in parsley called luteolin and brain health. Another study has shown an antidepressant effect. The next time the restaurant chef puts a sprig of parsley on your plate, don't brush it to the side. Eat it!

KICK UP THE VITAMIN K

Vitamin K's primary function is to help make a protein known as pro-thrombin, which is necessary for helping blood to clot. It also aids the body in making some other proteins for the blood, bones, and kidneys. And it may have another function: helping to prevent Alzheimer's. A 2016 study done at the University of North Carolina suggests that vitamin K affects calcium in the brain, which in turn lessens the risk of Alzheimer's.

Vitamin K is unique in that as well as being obtained from the diet, it is also made in the body from bacteria in the intestines. The prolonged use of antibiotics may affect your level of K because they destroy some bacteria in your intestines. If you're on antibiotics, it may make sense to supplement your vitamin K levels. There have been no reported problems in ingesting excess amounts of vitamin K, though moderation is always the best policy. Vitamin K has no established UL (upper limit).

Foods rich in vitamin K include wheat bran, wheat germ, beef liver, egg yolk, broccoli, cabbage, and green leafy vegetables, like turnip greens, spinach, and kale.

HIRE A PERSONAL TRAINER

Or at least *consult* a personal trainer. If you have trouble staying motivated, a personal trainer can be extremely beneficial. Having someone hold you accountable for your actions makes you more likely to do what you've said you were going to do. In addition to making sure you exercise regularly, a personal trainer can show you how to perform your workout for maximum advantage. Most gyms are staffed with people who will create the exercise regimen that's best for you and help you through it. The goal is to ensure that you are exercising correctly and at the proper pace. If you can afford a personal trainer, he or she will encourage you to commit to your routine and to push yourself just a wee bit harder—all of which is good for your brain. If you're not able to afford a trainer, then find a workout partner who can help serve the same purpose.

FALL IN LOVE

According to Dr. Frank Lawlis in his book *The IQ Answer*, falling in love stimulates your brain. "The act of loving someone can be directly observed through the brain and throughout your body. Your immune system sparkles with excitement that creates a better defense against disease, and you actually gain muscular strength. Your creativity soars from the stimulation of the right brain so that even males begin to integrate their intellectual vision with creativity." He notes that the type of love doesn't matter as much as the depth of feeling. "We know that newborn babies thrive when loved, while those without love tend to suffer in mental strengths.... [E]vidence indicates that those who love the most gain the greatest benefit cognitively." Research has shown that falling in love raises levels of nerve growth for a sustained period of time, perhaps as long as a year. The hormones produced apparently help to restore the nervous system and trigger new growth.

BITE SOME BLUEBERRIES

When it comes to brain protection, there's nothing quite like blueberries, which have been called the "brain berry." Blueberries contain antioxidant and anti-inflammatory compounds and may reverse short-term memory loss. In a study on reversing memory loss reported in *The Wall Street Journal*, blueberries had the strongest impact on the mental function of aging rodents than any of the other fruits tested. By eating only ½ cup of fresh or frozen blueberries a day you can receive their antioxidant protection and benefit from their anti-aging properties. When out of season buy them frozen to have in a smoothie. Or you can mix with yogurt and walnuts to create a delicious snack.

If you prefer your fruit fermented, here's some good news. Research at the University of Florida shows that blueberry wine has more antioxidants than white wine and most red wines. "For people seeking the potential health benefits of a glass of wine, blueberry wine is a comparable, and, in many instances, better alternative to grape wines," said Wade Yang, the lead researcher.

What this means for your health is a lower risk of heart disease, more vibrant and firmer skin, and a boost in brain power.

KNOW YOUR NUMBERS

When people think of their cholesterol levels, they're usually worried about their heart health. But high cholesterol is bad for your brain too. There's a well-established connection between high levels of cholesterol and the increased risk of stroke. New research suggests that high cholesterol is linked to Alzheimer's and other cognitive disorders. To keep your cholesterol on track, ask your doctor for a total lipoprotein profile so that you can be aware of not only your total cholesterol but also each component of your cholesterol. You may have a total cholesterol level that is desirable, but that doesn't mean your HDL (good) cholesterol and LDL (bad) cholesterol levels are in line. Your total cholesterol level will fall into one of three categories:

- Desirable: less than 200 mg/dL
- Borderline high risk: 200–239 mg/dL
- High risk: 240 mg/dL and over

If you have high cholesterol or other risk factors, your doctor will probably prescribe a cholesterol-lowering medication in combination with a healthy low-fat diet and exercise.

Having good levels of HDL is one of the most important factors in preventing ischemic strokes. These strokes occur when blood is blocked from flowing to the brain. Also, the less LDL you have, and the more HDL you have, the lower your risk for heart disease.

For HDL:
- Good: over 60 mg/dL
- Bad: less than 40 mg/dL

For LDL:
- Optimal: less than 100 mg/dL
- Near optimal: 100–129 mg/dL
- Borderline high: 130–159 mg/dL
- High: 160–189 mg/dL

TACKLE TRIGLYCERIDES

Triglycerides store fat, and too many of them in your blood signal a risk for heart attack and stroke. For your brain health, it's best to keep triglycerides at normal levels. They are measured as part of a full lipoprotein profile.

For triglycerides:

- Normal: less than 150 mg/dL
- Borderline high: 150–199 mg/dL
- High: 200–499 mg/dL
- Very high: 500 mg/dL or above

When it comes to trying to lower your LDL (bad) cholesterol and triglycerides, food choices are key. Foods that increase LDL also increase triglycerides. A combination of a diet low in saturated fat and cholesterol, regular physical activity, and a healthy weight can help you lower your total cholesterol as well as raise your HDL (good) cholesterol, lower your LDL, and lower your triglycerides. It is important to focus on your cholesterol intake as well as your saturated fat intake, which often occur together in foods. Cholesterol and most saturated fats come *only* from animal foods. Even though some foods of plant origin are high in fat or saturated fat, all plant foods are cholesterol free. Nuts, for example, are high in fat—mostly unsaturated fat—but are cholesterol free.

HAVE A HEART

Your heart and your blood vessels are responsible for transporting oxygen-rich and glucose-rich blood to all parts of the body. When impaired or damaged, your heart and your blood vessels can't get enough oxygen or glucose to the brain. So cardiovascular problems can lead to brain problems. Coronary heart disease is easier to prevent than it is to treat, especially if you have a family history of heart problems. The keys to keeping coronary heart disease at bay are regular, heart-strengthening exercise (at least four times a week) and maintaining a healthful diet that is low in fat and cholesterol and high in antioxidant-rich fruits and vegetables. Basically, a low-fat diet will have less animal protein, very little fried food, and increased amounts of whole grains and vegetables. Be good to your heart, and it will be good to your brain.

LOOK OUT FOR LEAD

Lead poses one of the greatest health threats. In high doses, this metal, which once was commonly used in household plumbing, can cause severe brain damage and even death. In low doses, it can cause nervous system damage in still-developing fetuses, infants, and children. Those most at risk are individuals living in homes constructed between 1910 and 1940, when lead service pipes were commonly used. Also risky are homes with plumbing consisting of copper pipes connected by lead-based solder (which was banned by federal law in 1986). Older chrome-plated bathroom fixtures, which are made of brass consisting of 3 to 8 percent lead, are also problematic. If you suspect your home may be subject to lead contamination, have it tested.

PILE ON THE GARLIC

Garlic lowers cholesterol levels, thins the blood, and boosts the immune system—all of which make for a happy and healthy brain. Garlic contains certain compounds that are known antioxidants and anti-inflammatories—there's a reason it's called a superfood. Recent research also suggests it may protect against Alzheimer's and Parkinson's, and that it may slow (or even reverse) damage from brain injury and environmental stresses.

Incorporate fresh garlic into salads by chopping, crushing, or putting it through a garlic press (two or three cloves a day is optimum). Whole garlic bulbs can be roasted in the oven, and the individual cloves can be squeezed out onto bread or toast as a creamy spread.

GET MORE POTASSIUM

Potassium is an electrolyte that works closely with its counterparts, chloride and sodium. Potassium helps regulate the flow of fluids and minerals in and out of the body's cells. It also sends oxygen to the brain, which lets the brain work better. Studies have shown that potassium may also reduce the risk of high blood pressure and stroke. Potassium is very important in converting blood sugar into glycogen, the storage form of blood sugar in your muscles and liver. This mineral is widely available in foods. Chronic diarrhea, vomiting, diabetic acidosis, kidney disease, or prolonged use of laxatives or diuretics could cause a deficiency. Most people excrete excess potassium in their urine. If the excess cannot be excreted—for instance, in the case of someone with kidney disease—it can cause heart problems. Some experts recommend a higher intake of potassium, around 3,500 milligrams per day, to help protect against high blood pressure.

A diet low in fat and cholesterol and rich in foods containing potassium, magnesium, and calcium—such as fruits, vegetables, legumes, and dairy foods—has shown evidence of reducing blood pressure. Potassium-rich foods include fresh meat, poultry, fish, figs, lentils, kidney beans, black beans, baked potatoes (with skin), avocados, orange juice, cantaloupes, bananas, and cooked spinach.

PLAY AN INSTRUMENT

According to Daniel G. Amen, MD, author of *Making a Good Brain Great*, the College Entrance Examination Board reported that students with experience in musical performance scored fifty-one points higher on the verbal part of the SAT and thirty-nine points higher on the math section than the national average. "It [learning to play a musical instrument] teaches the brain new patterns and stimulates wide areas of the cortex.... Learning a musical instrument, at any age, can be helpful in developing and activating temporal lobe neurons. As the temporal lobes are activated in an effective way, they are more likely to have improved function overall," Dr. Amen says. In another study Amen mentions, music majors were the most likely group of college grads to be admitted to medical school (66 percent, the highest percentage of any group).

JOG YOUR MEMORY

Memory is made and reinforced by the strength of connections between nerve cells and the formation of memory-storage protein molecules inside nerve cells. When a memory of a new idea is formed, like a name or an address, thousands of nerve cells are involved. If you don't use that bit of memory shortly after, it will soon fade away. But if you use it and reactivate the memory many times, you reinforce the stored chemical protein molecules that make up that memory. Reading these words creates thousands of electrochemical reactions in your brain. Often the brain is referred to as a computer, but the malleability and interactivity of the brain is far beyond any computer that is presently in use or on the horizon.

One way to challenge your brain is to work on improving your memory. Try memorizing lines of your favorite poems and see if you can recite them for the next seven days. Enhance your memorization at every opportunity and take advantage of the challenges life presents every day. For example, at social events, or whenever you are introduced to someone new, repeat the person's name to yourself three times and then use it in conversation. Meet as many people as possible, and then test yourself the next morning to see how many you can remember. Give yourself bonus points for remembering how they were dressed or what they did for a living.

TASTE THE RAINFOREST

Rainforest plants, while not as well known or as well studied as the herbs used in traditional Chinese and Indian medicines, contain many healing properties. You can learn more about them in the book *Kava: Medicine Hunting in Paradise* by Chris Kilham, who conducted research on medicinal plants around the world. In the meantime, here are some of the most important, as listed in the book *Herbal Secrets of the Rainforest* by Leslie Taylor:

- *Acerola.* Contains vitamin C. Promotes a healthy circulatory system—and your brain needs a healthy circulatory system!
- *Guarana.* Promotes health and energy.
- *Muira puama.* Relieves stress and promotes a healthy central nervous system.
- *Suma.* Aids in the regulation of cholesterol. Also used as a general health tonic. Also known as Brazilian ginseng.

Rainforests currently provide sources for one-quarter of today's medicines, and 70 percent of the plants found to have anticancer properties are found *only* in the rainforest. The rainforest and its immense undiscovered biodiversity hold the key to unlocking tomorrow's cures for devastating diseases. Put some rainforest into your life—it's good for your brain.

CAN THE SODA

The brain uses a large percentage of the body's glucose, but too much or too little glucose can have a detrimental effect on brain function. When you drink a can of soda, which contains ten teaspoons of table sugar, that sugar is absorbed into a bloodstream that usually only contains a total of four teaspoons of blood sugar. Your blood sugar level skyrockets, setting off alarms in the pancreas, and a large amount of insulin comes out to deal with the excess blood sugar. Some sugar is quickly ushered into the cells, including brain cells, and the rest is put into storage or into fat cells. When all this is done, maybe in about one hour, the blood sugar may fall dramatically and low blood sugar occurs. These rapid swings in blood sugar produce symptoms of impaired memory and clouded thinking. So think twice before swigging that soda—and don't assume artificially sweetened soda is better for you. Instead, try water or an herbal tea.

STIMULATE YOUR SENSES

In a recent interview, Dr. Stephen Brewer, medical director at the Canyon Ranch in Tucson, Arizona, suggested that it's important to find ways to stimulate your senses as a way to keep your brain active. Among other things, he suggested that you:

- Turn pictures in your house upside down; this will cause your brain to react and start mentally trying to put them the right way around again.
- Try dressing with your eyes closed.
- Leave cooked vanilla beans next to your bed to engage your sense of smell when you get up in the morning.
- Switch hands when brushing your hair or teeth from the one you usually use.
- Talk to yourself; one study suggested that this can improve your memory.

LEARN FIVE NEW WORDS

Like the athlete who takes time to warm up and flex his or her muscles before engaging in a strenuous activity, you can flex your brain cells with a few basic wordplay exercises to warm up your mental engine. Words are fun; they expand your mind. Pick up your dictionary and select five words you don't know. Commit their definitions to memory and write five sentences using them in different ways. See if you can recite their definitions from memory the next day. And then learn five more. If you're not in the habit of using your mind this way, acquiring a new vocabulary can be a challenge. However, practice makes perfect, and as you persevere, you'll soon discover that the task of committing words to memory will become increasingly easier to achieve and more satisfying.

MAKE ART

A recent study found that the creation of visual art, such as a painting or sculpture, improves effective interaction between different regions of the brain, particularly the frontal, posterior, and temporal brain regions. The participants in the study were a group of recent retirees who took a class in which they created paintings and drawings. The researchers stated that because of its positive effects on the brain, art making "may become an important prevention tool in managing the burden of chronic diseases in older adults." Creation of art, at any age, is also known to reduce stress, regardless of skill level.

PUT YOUR BRAIN ON CALCIUM

You know calcium helps build strong bones and teeth. What a lot of people don't know is that calcium is also important for brain functioning. Calcium provides links between important proteins that enable electrical signals within the brain. Without it, your brain would shut down.

Of course, calcium does a lot of other important things in your body. It works in conjunction with vitamin D, phosphorus, and fluoride to help promote strong and healthy bones. Vitamin D is necessary for the absorption of calcium in the body. Low levels of calcium intake can lead to osteomalacia (softening of the bones) and an increased risk of osteoporosis. Calcium has a UL (upper limit) set at 2,500 milligrams per day for adults and children. When consuming supplements up to this amount, no adverse effects are likely. However, higher doses over an extended period of time may cause kidney stones and poor kidney function as well as reduce the absorption of other minerals, such as iron and zinc.

Some of the best sources of calcium are foods in the dairy group, such as milk, cheese, and yogurt. In addition, some dark green leafy vegetables, such as broccoli, spinach, kale, and collards, are good sources. Other good sources include fish with edible bones, such as sardines and salmon, as well as calcium-fortified soymilk, tofu made with calcium, shelled almonds, cooked dried beans, calcium-fortified cereals, and calcium-fortified orange juice.

In a review of twenty-two studies, calcium supplementation was found to moderately reduce blood pressure in adults with hypertension, or high blood pressure, but had little effect on people with normal blood pressure. Take a minimum of 1,000 and a maximum of 2,000 milligrams a day. Experts recommend a two-to-one ratio of calcium to magnesium. If you regularly supplement with extra calcium, be sure to increase your magnesium intake too.

RECONSIDER RETIREMENT

You need to exercise your brain as if it were a muscle. You've heard the stories of the dangers of retiring without having a plan for how to fill your time. The stories are true, and the science is there to prove it. Most aspects of work, even the commute, the interaction with others, and the daily challenges, are stimulating. When you retire, if you don't build in challenges for your brain and body, then you can suffer physical and even mental decline. Studies also find that the more intellectually stimulating the job, the less likely it is that Alzheimer's will strike.

WRITE POETRY

It doesn't matter if you are really bad at writing poetry. In fact, that's precisely the reason to give it a try. Poetry is a creative form of writing that is indeed a fine art, but you don't have to master the form to earn benefits for your brain. Try your hand at various styles. You could write:

- An epic poem that celebrates, in a grand style, mythological and actual historical events.
- A narrative poem that tells a story in a somewhat simpler style. "Paul Revere's Ride" by the American poet Henry Wadsworth Longfellow is a narrative poem.
- An ode, which is a kind of lyric poem. An ode is a lyrical dedication to something or someone that the writer admires and loves. It describes how the subject of the ode affects the poet emotionally. Lyric poems are sensitive in tone. They express the poet's personal feelings of love, yearning, sorrow, and happiness.

Poetry can rhyme or not; poems that do not rhyme are referred to as blank verse. A great deal of poetry has a definite repetitive rhythm. Writing poetry will help you get in touch with your feelings, help you think metaphorically, and exercise your brain.

SEE A THERAPIST

Therapy is designed to alter the way you perceive your life and its challenges. A good therapist helps you put things in perspective, tame emotional mood swings, and reframe problems. As you learn to reframe, your brain gets happier and healthier. Having positive thoughts and taking positive actions bolster positive brain pathways and thus ultimately lead to improved brain function. Several studies have shown that cognitive therapy (i.e., talk therapy that teaches patients to counter negative thought patterns by replacing them with positive thoughts) can enhance brain function.

PRACTICE PILATES

Emphasizing the importance of the mind/body connection in attaining physical fitness, Joseph Pilates married critical elements of Eastern and Western philosophies to create what is known as the Pilates exercise program. Westerners approach health and fitness as a scientific task with a goal of maintaining and nurturing the body's muscles, bones, and circulatory and digestive systems. Eastern philosophies place much more importance on the development of mental and spiritual powers in the pursuit of pure health. Pilates students approach each movement with focus and determination, and they equally engage both body and mind in each physical endeavor. Pilates is a conditioning program designed to work the whole body—including your brain—simultaneously and uniformly. Joseph Pilates created his exercises with the intention "that each muscle may cooperatively and loyally aid in the uniform development of all our muscles. Developing minor muscles naturally helps to strengthen major muscles." As a result, every muscle is developed in every movement.

Studies have shown that after a mindful exercise such as Pilates or yoga, practitioners have better brain function. Because Pilates is similar to yoga, many of the benefits of yoga can be realized by performing Pilates exercises (for example, the stress-relieving aspect).

LIGHT A CANDLE

Smell is the most potent of all the senses because the information is delivered straight to your hypothalamus. Because moods, motivation, and creativity all stem from the hypothalamus, odors affect all of these processes. Think of a disgusting odor and how it can affect your appetite, or think of a fragrance that brings back a pleasant memory of a loved one, and you'll realize how intimately intertwined scents are with our emotions, memories, and ideas. Light a candle with a fragrance that invokes pleasant memories. Then lie back and soothe your hypothalamus.

HOP TO IT!

A thousand years ago brewers of English ale began using hops as a preservative. Much later they added it as an ingredient and discovered that their hops pickers suffered two peculiar effects: they tired quickly when working, and the female pickers got their menstrual periods earlier than normal. Science has since recognized the remarkable power of hops as a sedative. It has a calming effect on the body, soothes muscle spasms, relieves nervous tension, and promotes restful sleep. If you suffer from insomnia, make a tea with 1 teaspoon of dried hops in a cup of boiling water and drink it at bedtime. Capsules are also available. An old-fashioned cure for sleeplessness is to sleep on a small pillowcase filled with hops sprinkled with alcohol.

GO TO LECTURES

Lectures offer incredible opportunities to learn, acquire new interests, stay current, and improve your conversational skills. Pick challenging topics that you know nothing about—like neuroscience, archaeology, quantum physics, ancient history, or hieroglyphs—and charge up your brain cells by straining to understand. The more complex the subject matter, the more it will generate new thoughts and get your brainwaves sparking. Because your brain zooms into high gear when it tries to predict and understand what the speaker is saying, you'll stimulate parts of your brain that you don't just from reading. Think of the saying, "Listen with your brain, not your ears." The more you involve your whole brain in the process of engaging with a speaker, the better.

CHECK OUT CHICKEN

Red meat isn't great for your brain health but white meat—specifically, chicken—is great for your brain. Not only is it a good source of protein, it's also an excellent source of choline. No, no, not that stuff you put in the swimming pool to keep down the germs. Choline is used to make acetylcholine, a neurotransmitter that helps improve memory and brain function (it's also used in motor functions). It also helps regulate REM sleep, which is important for brain health. People with Alzheimer's have low levels of this neurotransmitter. There is some evidence that choline can serve a neuroprotective role. So broil up a little chicken and support your brain.

REVIEW YOUR WORK

Learning, as you may recall from your school days, involves understanding and memorization. As you become familiar with novel ideas, newly presented information, or a new vocabulary, your brain becomes much more receptive to retaining further knowledge—especially if you take the time to review and practice what you have already learned. It's a good idea, for example, to open your notebook and review any previously studied vocabulary before you turn to the next set of words. Your brain, like the rest of your body, is capable of achieving new skills.

COLOR! IT'S NOT JUST FOR KIDS

When you were young you probably had coloring books and crayons. Now more and more adults are discovering what fun it is to color—and it's also good for your brain.

Many therapists and psychologists recommend adult coloring books to their patients. Coloring stimulates the creative centers of the brain and staves off boredom, which is one of the principal causes of self-destructive behavior. Coloring is a calming activity that can help with conditions such as PTSD and chronic anger. It lets you sit quietly, concentrating on getting just the right shade of green or red on the picture in front of you while your mind relaxes. In a way, coloring is similar to meditation.

So next time you're near your local craft store, stop in and pick up an adult coloring book and some colored pencils. You'll be glad you did!

PICTURE THIS

Studies show that learning a new, complex skill can help prevent dementia. Researchers at the University of Texas at Dallas recently conducted a study testing the cognitive change for people who studied a challenging new skill, like learning how to use Photoshop, and compared how their brains fared against people who did enjoyable but nonchallenging activities like going to the movies. Those who spent significant time (about fifteen hours per week) learning about digital photography and image-editing software did much better on tests of memory. Those gains were kept even a year after the study ended. Researchers theorize that learning a complex task strengthens the connections between neurons in the brain—unlike games, such as crossword puzzles, which only have a limited effect on short-term memory.

TAKE A NATURE BREAK

If your idea of camping is a hotel without room service, we've got news for you: your brain needs you to go camping. Being out in nature—not just looking at it from your car window, but actual toes-in-the-grass being in nature—works wonders for your brain. And we're not just talking a fifteen-minute break with the pigeons in the park before you head back to your cubicle. We're talking a weekend away from your cell phone and your cares.

Recent research has shown that not only does time spent in nature help you de-stress, it actually helps your brain function better. People who spent three days backpacking in natural surroundings did 50 percent better on a test of creativity than people who left their gear in the garage.

Even if you can't get away from it all you can get away from it some, and that will still help your brain. Researchers at the University of Exeter Medical School analyzed data to find that people who lived near green space (even just a park) were less likely to have depression, migraines, and anxiety than people who did not. Researchers suspect that being out in nature helps your brain primarily by lowering stress hormones in your body. One researcher speculates that because we evolved in nature, we naturally relax once we are back in nature. It turns out that one of the best ways to boost your happiness is to hit the trails.

TAKE A DAY OFF

Numerous surveys of American workers show they rarely take time off for vacations, and when they do, they're constantly checking email and texts from work anyway. This is a great way to burn out your brain. One study showed that people who took off one day per week—one day without any work-related tasks—ended up being more productive overall than those who didn't. Not surprisingly, they also reported feeling less stressed. One researcher analyzing data from several studies found that idleness—not having to do anything work-related—helped the brain process information, make new connections, and even understand ourselves and other people better (one benefit of idleness is introspection). We also solve problems and remember things better if we take real breaks from work.

TUNE OUT FROM TV

Your mom probably told you that television rots your brain. She was right. Studies have shown a link between children watching television and more aggressive behavior, and other studies have shown a correlation between television viewing and obesity. And a recently completed longitudinal study showed that watching television makes us dumber. Researchers followed a group of young adults who were all around age twenty-five and monitored their viewing habits. Twenty-five years later, the ugly truth was confirmed. People who watched the most television—more than three hours a day—scored the worst on brain tests.

Another study, this of younger children, showed that television viewing was associated with poorer verbal ability. Television viewing has also been shown to disrupt sleep cycles—and the poorer your sleep, the greater your memory and other cognitive problems. For children, concerns include delayed mental development and the increased likelihood of developing attention deficit hyperactivity disorder. People who watch a lot of television also have less social connection with others, and social connection is one of the things that contributes to brain health.

Need more convincing that it's high time to ditch the satellite dish? Yet another study showed that unhappy people watch the most television. The opposite was true of other activities. For example, for people who liked to read, the more they read, the happier they were. For television watchers, the more they watched, the unhappier they were. In other words, if you want to be happy, dump the television.

HACK JOURNAL

Hack	Date	Notes

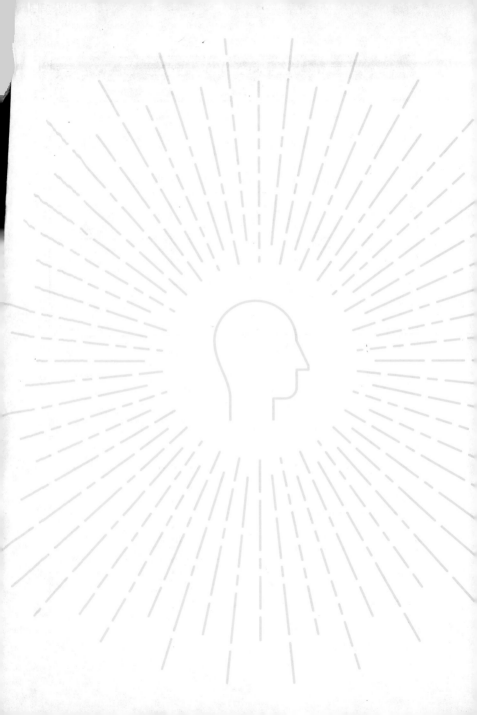